D1561887

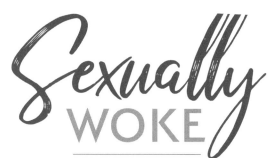

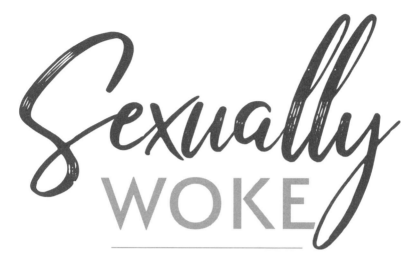

Sexually WOKE

Awaken the Secrets to Your Best Sex Life in Midlife & Beyond

Dr. Susan Hardwick-Smith, OB/GYN

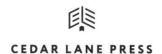

CEDAR LANE PRESS

Published in the United States by Cedar Lane Press, LLC
Lancaster, Pennsylvania

Paperback ISBN: 978-1-950934-44-7
E-book ISBN: 978-1-950934-45-4
Audio book ISBN: 978-1-950934-71-3

Library of Congress Control Number: 2020942577
Printed in the United States of America

10 9 8 7 6 5 4 3 2

Cedar Lane Press
PO Box 5424
Lancaster, PA 17606-5424
www.CedarLanePress.com

To learn more about Cedar Lane Press books, or to find a retailer near you, email Info@CedarLanePress.com or visit us at www.CedarLane-Press.com.

DEDICATION

*To Liam, Isabel, and Lily, who taught me how to love unconditionally.
To Taranatha, my father, who bought me the Dharma. To my sister Liz,
whose death showed me how to live, the courage to be my best Self,
and the example of how to love with an undefended heart.*

CONTENTS

Why Does the World— and You— Need This Book?

The end of my life in a trance was on a Sunday morning in March 2014. I woke up from a dream. It wasn't just any dream; it was an extraordinary, happy dream of being completely whole and making passionate love with my true soul mate. Still damp with perspiration from a night of hot flashes, I bolted awake, sat up, and proclaimed defiantly and joyously, "I don't have to do this anymore!"

My then-husband stirred in half-sleep and mumbled, "What?"

What, indeed. Was I still dreaming? The voice seemed to have spoken through me from a higher source. "Nothing," I replied and then headed downstairs to brew a cup of tea.

Yes, that was the end of my life in a trance—because once you wake up, you can never go back to a numb, robotic sleep.

Weeks later, I mustered the courage to leave my 18-year relationship, marking both one of the hardest and easiest things I've ever done. Hard, because turning lives upside down caused a lot of temporary suffering for a lot of people. Easy, because I felt like I had no other choice. The life force inside me was directing the way, despite the short-term cost.

Then came my aha moment—a true spiritual awakening—about the questions that had percolated silently for years as I'd watched and listened to my gynecologic patients struggle with midlife. What was the connection between a woman's sex drive as we age and the degree of relationship intimacy and spirituality? Why did my sex drive come back with a passion post-divorce? Why had so many of my patients experienced the same, whether tied to a new perspective of an existing committed relationship or at the onset of a new one? What did spiritual connectedness and sex have in common? Could the dots be connected? *Could I connect the dots?*

Around the time of midlife, women face what feels like the perfect storm as our meticulously arranged lives start to unravel. Disappearing fertility brings with it the stark realization of our own mortality. Personal illnesses or physical limitations may set in. Our bodies are changing in ways that can be devastating to accept. That voice in our heads questions our relevance, even if we have no desire for childbearing, asking, "If I'm not fertile, then who am I? Am I officially old now?" (I didn't know whether to laugh or cry when I received an introductory mail offer from AARP right after my 50th birthday.) Our children are often struggling or leaving; aging parents may be sick or dying. Relationships are changing, and our careers are either as far as they will go or coming to an end. Combine these forces with a raging storm of hormonal change, and we are standing at a fork in the road. We have a choice. Either wake up, accept, and embrace the wondrous possibilities of this new reality or pile on more delusion and denial.

Like most of my patients, I had been stuck in the latter until I suddenly—literally overnight—became intensely aware of the optimism and hope that had been a giant blind spot for me. Instead of seeing the second half of life as an end to everything I valued, I sensed a vast openness of limitless possibility and freedom from the endless hamster wheel that had occupied most of my previous life.

This is an idea worth talking about. After more than 20 years as an expert in women's health, I can tell you with absolute certainty that most of us are missing out on this great truth and the hope it offers: our best life, including our sexual life, doesn't have to end at 50, 60, or 70. The truth is, it has the potential to grow richer and fuller with every moment we're blessed to be alive.

Back to the Beginning

When I was growing up, discussing sex was off-limits. Even saying the word s-e-x was an offense that would get me sent to my room, which turns out not to be the ideal strategy for stamping out sexual behaviors in teenagers.

You might remember that '70s book *The Joy of Sex*. One of my older sisters somehow snagged a copy from a progressive friend's parents, and my early sex education happened while hidden under the covers in my bedroom, poring over the peculiar pencil drawings of what was intended to represent a regular 1970s couple. Visions of that chubby bearded man and his partner with hairy armpits still pop up at inopportune times.

Fast-forward 35 years to our current world with unlimited access to seeing people having sex, and most of us are still under the covers with our fears and shame. There are few places for real, open conversations about sexuality, particularly in what I politely call our "middle years." As the leader of a sizable, all-female obstetrics and gynecology medical practice, thousands of intimate accounts of intense suffering and confusion about midlife have been told to me behind closed exam room doors. My office became a literal sacred place where all the things women are most afraid to say have permission to come out without fear of judgment.

This was all just super interesting in a detached way, like studying a disease you don't have, until I personally started to experience the menopause process at age 47. I began to hear my own intensely private story being mirrored back daily by my patients, and I realized I had nothing much to offer other than empathy and a hormone prescription. Sadly, and more importantly, each of my patients felt alone and thought there was something wrong with her. Why weren't we sharing this stuff with each other or our life partners?

It's ironic, really. In this age of information overload, women of all ages, particularly 40–65, are often in the dark about what's happening to our bodies and have few resources to share when it comes to our changing sexual beings.

> In this age of information overload, women of all ages, particularly 40–65, are often in the dark about what's happening to our bodies and have few resources to share when it comes to our changing sexual beings.

beings. I remember a book quietly slipped to me by my parents at around age 12 titled *What's Happening to Me?* And that was it. No conversation. Menopause felt like *What's Happening to Me? Part II*. Once again, information was slipped privately, primarily through clandestine whispers and rumors but rarely from reliable sources. Our mothers often either forgot or denied that menopause ever happened to them. Even close friends would hesitate to reveal the truth, choosing to hide behind the myth that everything was okay, while others would create humor around the suffering to avoid facing it head on.

As it turns out, when you start a conversation about something private, potentially embarrassing, shameful, and controversial, the last place you want to look is at yourself, but it was inevitable. I started talking to women my age about sex, which you might think is normal at the gynecologist's office. But trust me, most physicians dedicate about 10 minutes to each patient and are generally hoping to scoot out the door before the sexuality topic comes up. Most of us have no idea what to say. And we sure don't want to look in the mirror and face what is dissatisfying in our own lives and relationships. But something told me this was work that really needed to be done, and I began investigating and learning for the first time what was really going on. It's amazing what I learned just by deeply listening and mustering the courage to look honestly at myself.

Most of the stories I heard from patients weren't pretty. My own story certainly wasn't. At 45, I had been with the same guy for 18 years, married for 12, given birth to three kids within 19 months—you do the math—and we had two big careers. Our sex life had been on life support for years; it was something we did not and could not talk about. I rationalized that it was normal because of the kids, our work schedules, my changing hormones, and nature's obvious plan—trust me, I'm a doctor, so I know nature's plan—that went along with the biological impossibility and/or loss of desire for future fertility.

Like so many patients, I had intellectualized and rationalized my sex life into one of the deepest corners of my mind. You know the place: where all the best secrets stay hidden so you can't hear them, as if your hands are over your ears while you chant la-la-la. I conveniently rationalized and consoled many women, I'm ashamed to admit, by explaining that when your body knows you can't get pregnant, biology tells you that you don't need to have sex. In reality, this is just a doctor's excuse for not being turned on anymore, and I had plenty of patients in the same boat every day to make me feel safe and silently supported. In sharing my own story, I connected with many, many patients who felt the same way, and we all breathed a collective sigh of relief about not being alone after all.

Whew! We were normal! But normal wasn't necessarily optimal. Very few of us were happy about our waning sex lives, and many of us were straight up miserable. Not to mention our partners.

Case in point, my marriage was going downhill fast. We stopped talking. We stopped looking at each other. We stopped connecting, and my sex drive was below zero. I stopped caring where he was or what he was doing and only wanted him home to cover childcare. My patients' marriages were going downhill too. This downhill epidemic spoke true to a startling statistic: divorce rates for women over 50 have doubled since 1990 while the overall divorce rate has declined. What's going on here?

> As I dug deeper, I met other angels from widely varied backgrounds, races, and religions. Despite their differences, they had a whole lot in common. This was the gold I was looking for.

Just as my sex life was in the tank, at least one patient near my age would bounce into the office every week with a rosy glow and stories of a sex life that blew the lid off my old hippy book. I listened wide-eyed as if talking to an angel delivering an important message. I joked with some of these lucky angels that I wanted to draw their blood and find out what genetic mutation they carried so I could sell it, and then they could visit me on my private island. But it was easier than that because some surprising patterns began to emerge.

First, many of these women had a new partner. Don't get me wrong; I'm not advocating that a new partner is your only hope, although it does remain one of the most reliable options. Thankfully, for those of us who want to keep our current partner, I also met and studied a different group of women near my age with a self-reported vibrant sex life and a deep sense of well-being and connection with their long-term mate. These ladies generally reported having a profoundly new relationship with a long-term partner, often through counseling after a crisis or a very intentional process of reconnection, shedding harmful old habits and creating healthier new ones. It wasn't an accident, and it was rarely easy. As I dug deeper, I met other angels—some in partnerships, some single, some gay—from widely varied backgrounds, races, and religions. Despite their differences, they had a whole lot in common. This was the gold I'd been looking for.

These women shared an unusual level of self-awareness and were comfortable in their own skins, inevitably through some process of self-discovery and healing old wounds. Beyond a connection with their partner, they were deeply connected to themselves. They felt whole and were in a relationship—or not—out of conscious choice, not fear or compulsion.

Channeling one of my favorite books of all time, Shel Silverstein's *The Missing Piece Meets the Big O*, they had mastered rolling along without another piece to fill some bottomless psychic hole. These women had filled it themselves. They knew their own bodies, were unashamed, knew how to pleasure themselves, and were comfortable asking for—even demanding—what they needed. They knew how to communicate with kindness and truth, and seemed to have accepted themselves as being enough, loving themselves first with the understanding that you can't give what you don't have.

An important spiritual element was also a common factor in all of these angels' lives, be it through God, yoga, meditation, nature, or conscious generosity practices. These women shared a deep understanding of their connection to something bigger than themselves that was based in love, connection, and compassion.

Confirming recent research in the #MeToo movement, more than one-fourth of them had suffered sexual trauma, and all had struggled in numerous other ways. They were not innately lucky. Life hadn't been handed to them on a silver platter, but they had found a way to make lemonade out of lemons—or perhaps to see lemonade where I saw lemons. They had moved from a position of victimhood, where the world happens to me—to a place of creativity and strength, where the world happens by me. They were not perfect, and all had bad days. They were works-in-progress that hadn't arrived anywhere magical; rather they were on a path, arriving every day exactly where they were and actively committing to being present in the moment.

Most fascinating to me was that these women reported amazingly vibrant and fulfilling sex lives, which presented in many different ways. But all of them said that sex, or their relationship with sex and with their bodies, was better than ever. They saw the second half of life as an opportunity, not a curse. They approached their relationships with themselves and their partners with intention and found ways to keep things fresh, new, and fun.

Wow! If it was possible for them, then hopefully it was possible for me, and perhaps I could teach it to others.

From Doom to Optimism

Quite suddenly my perspective changed from viewing midlife as a frightening black hole of doom and gloom to a source of great optimism and excitement. There was hope for us after all, and perhaps together we could find a better way to relate to this second half of life.

Since references to "awakening" and "waking up" came up so often in my interviews, I began to refer to my angels in the same way that one of my patients referred to herself: "Sexually Woke."

So after years of telling myself (and unfortunately also telling my patients) that declining libido and loss of our sexual selves is a normal part of the biology of female midlife, I had to face the fact that I was dead wrong. This took some time to accomplish since I had built my life around never being wrong. As a scientist, I'd been trained to think that I should know the answer to everything, that everything real can be measured, and that traditional medicine was infallible. My mind had to shift from the world of certainty to the world of curiosity and letting go of being right.

If women aged 40 to 65—and older—can have the joyful sexual energy of a 22- year-old then clearly nothing is gone; it's just hidden. And that means we can find it.

My own midlife career crisis slapped me in the face as I realized traditional medicine was spending billions of dollars every year to make people physically "healthy" with "numbers" that were brag-worthy. But the very same "healthy" patients often remained disconnected, depressed, and surrounded by dysfunctional relationships, repressed feelings, and resentment. Doctors seemed more interested in a patient's vital signs and lab results than her whole sense of physical, emotional, and spiritual wellness. As a patient myself, I was accustomed to hearing from a doctor, "Congratulations, you are just fine!" when my heart was telling me loud and clear that I was most definitely not fine. Unfortunately, no one wanted to talk about what was really not fine. For sure that would take longer than 10 minutes, and there was no pill to fix it.

Part of me was suffocated, stuck in a box, and not expected to complain. I was, after all, an "older woman" and largely irrelevant in our culture that glorifies youth. I'd been told my whole life that sex was something men wanted and women either succumbed to sex or used it as currency in exchange for something else. Being outspoken about sex or what I needed sexually was not feminine and certainly was not acceptable, especially "at my age." I wanted to be whole. I wanted to connect. I wanted to feel my feelings. I wanted someone to see me and truly listen to me. I wanted to have sex—lots and lots of sex—but just not the kind I was having, and not with the person I was having it with. The sexually woke were my saviors and my inspiration. If women aged 40 to 65—and older—can have the joyful sexual energy of a 22-year-old, then clearly nothing is gone; it's just hidden. And that means we can find it. So I set out on a mission to create the map to rediscover it.

My mission quickly led to an intense grief about my own loss, as well as a flood of empathy and compassion for the losses of so many of us—the loss of one of the potentially greatest sources of connection in our lives and arguably (literally, really) the source of the life-force itself. This is not to say that those not engaging in sexual activity due to conscious choice or circumstance cannot truly be happy, because of course they can. In fact, some of the most deeply content and connected people I have met and interviewed are not sexually active in the traditional sense. But I do believe there needs to be a deep connection to the ever-present sexual, emotionally fertile, and generative part of our being to live as our full, authentic selves.

The Feminine Sexual Being

Here's something that I have learned to be certain of through my own experience. The vitally important sexual part of our being exists in every person. She is creative, energetic, connected, generous, free, and too often hidden. She is intimately aware of her physical feelings, as well as her emotions and where they show up in her body. She doesn't just have sex. She makes love, both with her partner and herself—if her lifestyle supports that—and more importantly, with the world. Making love with the world is showing up in your integrity, in other words: integrated, pulled together, complete, and whole as your full, unashamed self, and operating from a place where everything belongs. Wrinkles, soft belly, sagging boobs, gray hair, and all. That's sexy. And if it doesn't sound like you, don't worry; you are not alone.

She's in there, patiently waiting to be found. This book will hopefully help you find her. Denying that we are a sexual being at any age is denying our wholeness. Our sexual being is a huge part of our complete, authentic self. Cutting off part of ourselves by definition limits us from reaching our full potential. And at the risk of over-dramatization, reaching our full potential seems to be the purpose of life.

> Denying that we are a sexual being at any age is denying our wholeness. Our sexual being is a huge part of our complete, authentic self.

Waking up to who we really are and reconnecting in the deepest spiritual sense with ourselves, our partners (if we have one), and the world is the beautiful potential wisdom of midlife. We can finally be free to find ourselves and show up as we are, unashamed. This often comes after a lifetime of serving the needs of others and following a path that was not our own. My work became a calling, focused on blowing the lid off this taboo hiding place of shame, secrets, and lies, and starting a conversation about what's really going on. Together, I hoped we could figure out how to embody a life that mirrors our fully integrated and innately sexy potential.

Getting Down to Business: The Study

That calling led me to undertake one of the largest studies ever done on this subject, involving more than 1,000 women ages 40–65 who were surveyed extensively about the most intimate parts of their sexual, spiritual, and relational lives. I titled it the "Midlife, Relationships, and Sex Study" and will refer to it as MRS going forward. (Please read this in your head as three individual letters—M-R-S—not "Mrs."—to avoid associating this only with married women!).

Many brave participants agreed to share their stories through recorded interviews and written testimonies. Through this enormous shared body of information, I was able to document the truth behind my suspicions tied to years of personal and professional experience and to describe with statistics what is common and "normal." To my delight, I was also able to investigate the lives of women who seemed to have found the "secrets" to living a vibrant, connected, and passionate second half of life.

Moment of Gratitude

Stepping back for a second, it's from a position of great privilege that we can even consider having a great sex life. I will forever remember hearing in middle school that Marie Antoinette could not understand why the masses of Parisians were rebelling because they didn't have any bread, and she allegedly suggested, "Let them eat cake." While this story is likely untrue, it's a great example of unconscious privilege, ignorance, and bias that can exist in each of us.

I am extremely conscious that most women in the world have more pressing things to worry about than fulfilling sex. If you are privileged enough to be able to read, to have lived past 40, to have the means to have bought this book, and to care about improving your sex life, I invite you to pause right now for a few moments of gratitude. It's only in recent recorded history that we've been able to evolve beyond the human brain's primary biological drive to survive and to consider, instead, how to thrive. Pursuing happiness is a privilege that we should never forget; it's a luxury that comes after survival is taken for granted.

> Pursuing happiness is a privilege that we should never forget; it's a luxury that comes after survival is taken for granted.

My own story has clearly influenced this book, and I am happy to share it in these pages. How a small-town girl from New Zealand ended up in Houston, Texas, growing the largest all-female obstetrics and gynecology practice in the country; developing women's health programs in rural Africa; traveling a spiritual path that took me through divorce and a brutal custody battle; and then finding (and losing) my best friend and my first deeply connected lover at age 47—is certainly a testament to the power of having a deep faith that I could do hard things.

Deeply knowing you can do hard things is foundational for happiness and comes from—guess what?—a history of doing hard things and surviving. No one gets through life unscathed, nor should we want to, since it is the experience of struggle, failure, and survival that teaches us to be brave and to have the courage to keep trying.

The Invisible Thread

The connecting thread in everything I have pursued is a genuine love of people, a passionate desire for connection, and a deeply rooted understanding that *there is more here than meets the eye.*

We live in a world where experiences skate across the surface of a vast, deep ocean. As a self-described seeker, I'm pulled to go deeper and refuse to live an unlived and unexamined life. Parenting, leadership, writing, speaking, and even competing in crazy-sounding athletic activities like Ironman triathlons have forced me to connect with my own inner potential in the face of plenty of failure. One thing I know for sure is that we are all capable of so much more than we are taught to believe. If we are not failing often enough, we are not pushing up against the edges of our potential.

Most importantly in the context of this book, I mustered the courage to leave my first marriage and pursue a life of connection and authenticity. This led me to be available to find true love and to commit to living and loving with an undefended heart. Equally important, I sought and found a group of deeply intimate female friends on similar paths from all over the world. Transformation simply cannot take place in an echo chamber.

The wisdom of midlife gave my patients and me the strength to say "F&*# it." I am ready to find out and be who I was put on this earth to be; I have nothing to lose except the last half of my life in the prison of living someone else's dream. The playing field opened up into an endless space of possibility. No labels, no agendas and no stereotypes—just a blank canvas on which to find the emerging picture of what was there all along: my best Self, my fully realized potential.

> Equally important, I sought and found a group of deeply intimate female friends on similar paths. Transformation simply cannot take place in an echo chamber.

My recent passion for studying midlife sexuality blossomed as I navigated the same stormy waters that my patients described. We are all truly in the same boat, on the planet, as women, as humans facing aging and with sexuality. As American Buddhist nun Pema Chodron writes, "Compassion is not a relationship between the healer and the wounded. It's a relationship between equals. Only when we know our own darkness—can we be present with the darkness of others. Compassion becomes real when we recognize our shared humanity."

As a traditionally trained doctor, my jaw dropped the first time I read this quote. My eyes were opened to a magnificent new level of connection when I changed my perspective from a "healer-wounded" or "hero-victim" relationship when caring for patients. While I have additional training and more medical expertise than my patients, deep down we are all just women. And in midlife, we are all going through remarkably similar things. You don't need to have cancer to be an oncologist, but it would probably help. Going through menopause as a gynecologist was the perfect way for me to truly empathize and connect with what my patients had been describing all those years.

> Going through menopause as a gynecologist was the perfect way for me to truly empathize and connect with what my patients had been describing all those years.

My fascination with connection exploded after years of feeling the icy cold of its absence and then finally understanding the transformative power of connection in my first deeply intimate relationship at the young age of 47. Perhaps studying sexuality was the Holy Grail for my lifelong fascination with connection, for what greater connection exists than that of truly loving sex?—or, more accurately, truly loving intimate physical connection. Our sexuality is expressed in so many more ways than just vaginal intercourse.

The Path to Connection and Satisfaction

In the coaching world, we frequently ask clients to examine and describe their current state, fully accept where they are, and then create a vision for an ideal state, which we create stepping stones to work toward. Following that path, this book is divided into three parts. Part One discusses the art and science of midlife sexuality to get us off on the same foot with some basic knowledge. Part Two looks at where we are now, how we got here, and where we might want to be. Part Three lays out a roadmap of how to get there based on the experiences of real women, including me, who are on the journey and want to share it.

No longer the secret knowledge of a few outliers, this path to deep sexual connection and satisfaction is available to anyone who is ready to commit and is willing to embark on the journey. With deep gratitude for my own awakening, the courage to let go of old, limiting beliefs, and uprooting my old life in the hope of finding my true Self, I am now on that path too.

What I have to offer through my education, experience, and observations is really not my story; it's our story. What one of us feels, most of us feel. What one of us experiences, most of us experience. My hope is that the information you find here will help you feel less alone and more part of this great international sea of women connected by our common humanity. Together we are embracing the desire to be fulfilled, to love, and be loved, to see and be seen, and to believe that transformation is possible.

The names of women interviewed for this book have been changed to honor their privacy, and some interviews have been edited or combined.

"In out-of-the-way places of the heart,
Where your thoughts never think to wander,
This beginning has been quietly forming,
Waiting until you were ready to emerge."

—*John O'Donohue*

THE ART AND SCIENCE OF MIDLIFE SEXUALITY

ONE

The MRS Study and What's "Normal"

If your early sex education was anything like mine, you might have missed some important information. I am constantly amazed at how little most adult women know about how our bodies function. Our culture sets us up to believe that certain revered people, especially doctors and celebrities, know all there is to know about women's health, including about how to navigate the changes of midlife. The problem is that assumption is dead wrong. All of us, including the "experts" that we look to, are victims of what we have been taught, and few of us are operating from real science or experience. For the most part, we believe what we are told. And much of what we are told is just not true.

Doctors Are People Too

Even in medical school, information about sexuality was limited to a day or two of discussion. Our sex education included some anatomic mechanical description of the reproductive system and the various ways it could fail. After all, since we were training to be doctors, we were learning about sickness, not wellness. Most excitingly, we were shown a variety of pornographic movies, including male and female masturbation, heterosexual and homosexual sex, and "elderly sex" (with actors close to my current age). These movies were designed to ensure that these mostly inexperienced and rather nerdy 20-something medical students had at least a small clue about what our patients were doing, particularly since most of us weren't doing much of it at all.

I remember the sex movies as being the unofficial highlight of the first year of medical school. After hearing the second-year students giggle and tease us about it, many of the older students ditched their own classes to come back and watch the famous movies again. For probably half the class, this was their only sexual experience involving other people. In the anatomy lab, discussion and dissection of the sexual organs brought on the same nervous joking that you probably remember from middle school health class.

Suffice it to say, the idea that your doctor knows more about sex than you or is more experienced or comfortable talking about it than you is most likely false. If you saw the level of nerdiness, inexperience, and body discomfort in my medical school class, you would be wise to not expect much help around sex when you visit your doctors.

Believe it or not, even four years of OB/GYN residency taught me almost nothing about female sexuality. Most OB/GYN teaching programs serve young, underserved populations and focus on pregnancy. Gynecology for mature populations focuses on surgery. There was absolutely no discussion about taking care of the whole woman throughout her lifespan. We were taught to focus strictly on the part of the body between the belly button and the external genitalia. Maybe the breasts too, but that's it. Everything else was someone else's problem. The truth is the so-called experts most of us turn to for advice about sexuality have very little idea how to help and are probably searching on Google just like you.

Hey, I am no different than anyone else. I remember being sure in elementary school that boys had cooties and in high school that you could get pregnant any day of the month. That's what I was taught. Maybe my teachers thought it was true, or maybe it was clever manipulation to create fear around sex. When I found out as an adult that getting pregnant could only happen on a few days of every month at most, I was completely baffled and felt like I had been lied to. Apart from that, I had no clue why I bled every month or how the pills and IUD that I later used even worked. I just believed. That kind of blind faith not only rids us of our ability to make educated choices but also leaves us completely confused about what's happening as our bodies change.

What's Wrong with Me?

Many times, when I was up to my ears in data, sticky notes, and transcribed interviews, I wondered why on earth I took on a massive yearlong research project after 20 years in private practice with retirement in sight. Honestly, I think it points to the degree of my desperation with not only the lack of information but also the lies and cultural ignorance that my patients and I were faced with as we matured.

Western culture seems to be systematically set up to make us feel not good enough. When it comes to midlife sexuality, there is not enough therapy, plastic surgery, Botox, or hormone replacement in the world to fix what's "wrong." With the forces of social media and reality TV fueling the fire by feeding us details about everyone else's "perfect" lives, no wonder we feel alone.

In fact, one of the most common presenting complaints in my office is some version of "something is wrong with me." At a doctor's office, one might think this is expected since you don't usually go to the doctor unless something is wrong. But in women's health, I can honestly say that about 50 percent of my patients' problem visits are for issues that fall within the normal range of human experience. Our culture expects you to always feel great, look great, smell great, be symmetrical, and have no itches, tingles, discharges, stings, aches, or other discomforts. If something doesn't feel good or something isn't working perfectly, something must be wrong. This might be the single most harmful myth that you've ever been fed.

If something doesn't feel good or something isn't working perfectly, something must be wrong. This might be the single most harmful myth that you've ever been fed.

Since few of us talk about our sexuality openly and common information sources are sketchy to say the least, you might be stuck in a place of isolation and feeling as if you're the only one with something wrong. I can tell you that when my life started unraveling in my mid-40s, I was pretty certain that everyone else's sex life was better than mine, everyone else's marriage was happy, everyone else was financially secure, and everyone else's kids were always well-behaved and unconditionally loving. That's how it looked on Facebook anyway.

Phew! Struggling Is Normal

The fact is human experience is defined by discomfort. One of the most important lessons I have ever learned came from Eastern spiritual wisdom. In Buddhist terms, life naturally comes with inevitable unsatisfactoriness or difficulty. You get what you don't want, and you don't get what you do want. Things that you don't like stick around longer than you want, and things you love leave or die. That should be expected. Expecting that everything should be perfect is delusional.

Your body changes in sometimes unwanted ways as you get older. When you get up in the morning, you have bad breath. Teenagers can provide seven years of intermittent misery for their parents. If you live in a city, traffic is a reality that can't be avoided. If you are woman, you will have 35 or more years of monthly bleeding, which is a pain to say the least. You will get sick, old, and then die. Everything and everyone you love will disappear or die as well. This is all normal. If that makes you think that I am being pessimistic or depressing, it's because our culture teaches us not to talk about these things. But they are real. Can we dare to be real?

The problem isn't that we suffer. The problem is that we resist the reality of suffering and get stuck in aversion by pushing away the realities we don't like and trying to fix and cling to pleasant things that will inevitably change. Being at constant battle with "what is" and denying the reality of impermanence is exhausting, fruitless, and in many spiritual circles is understood to be the primary cause of stress or suffering. Understanding this is really hard and really useful.

As a doctor, I am in the caring and compassion business, which comes with a genuine wish to end suffering and a commitment to take action to alleviate suffering when I can. So the suggestion isn't to give up caring for the suffering of ourselves and others, but to start from a place of acceptance rather than denial and do what we can from there. There's the suffering you can't avoid, like old age, bodily changes, and death. There's also the suffering you can avoid, like fighting or denying the fact that it's happening. In spiritual circles, this is sometimes called the "second arrow," and it can hurt more than the first one.

Let me give you an example. Recently I strained my lower back lifting weights. The back pain hurt a little. Most of the time I didn't even notice it, but the worst part was my story about the pain. Maybe I would not be

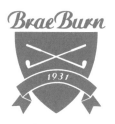

BraeBurn Country Club Ladies Association Harmonious Hormones

March 8, 2022

Hors d'oeuvres

Gazpacho Shooter
Mini crab cake

Soup

Red Lentil
Paprika olive oil

Entrée

Sesame Crusted Tuna
Pan seared ahi tuna, quinoa and kale salad,
Toasted peanuts, Thai chili vinaigrette

Dessert

Acai Berry Sorbet

able to work out for a week, and I would gain weight. Or maybe I would never be able to run again. Maybe there was something really wrong with my back and it would be the beginning of the end of my athletic life. As it turns out, my back was fine in a few days. The physical injury itself was nothing compared to the mental suffering that I added with my aversion to the pain. That's the second arrow.

Accepting suffering doesn't mean giving up. Far from it. It means opening up. The suggestion is not to accept whatever suffering comes your way like a doormat, rather it is to accept your own experience of it. That's totally different. If you have cancer, or if you are in a miserable marriage, accepting your experience does not mean avoiding seeking help. It means accepting and being present with your own emotions and experiences, and allowing them in rather than fighting them off or inflaming them with your mind. Do you ever deny your suffering and state that you are fine, or do you go the opposite way and create an imaginary disaster out of what may be a small and temporary inconvenience (like my back pain)? Unless you're being chased by a tiger, accept first, act later. This allows us to act from love and clarity rather than from denial and reactivity.

> Everyone, including me, seemed to believe some similar version of "something is wrong with me." But how is it possible that a similar thing is wrong with everyone? Logically, this just didn't make sense.

If we agree that the appropriate and wise response to suffering is compassion, then how about we give ourselves some? Rather than covering our ears or beating ourselves up, how about giving others and ourselves a real or metaphorical hug? Maybe we can make it better and maybe we can't, but let's start with the acceptance that we are suffering. How about, "Dear Self: Ouch! That must be really hard. I understand," instead of "Just suck it up, you big baby, and don't look so weak!" (my favorite) or "OMG, I think I'm going to die!"

Have you lost the ability to talk about your suffering and believe you're the only one struggling? Do you think struggling is synonymous with weakness or deficiency, or that if you were doing things right or had the right partner or the right (fill in the blank)—things should be easy? I can't think of another field in which this almost universal delusional thinking is expressed more strongly than sexuality. I am not judging. We all have delusional thinking. All of us tell stories to ourselves that are inconsistent with "what is."

As a gynecologist, I had the rare experience of seeing my own delusion expressed by the huge number of patients I saw every year who felt exactly the same things, albeit in deeply unique and personal ways. Everyone, including me, seemed to believe some similar version of "something is wrong with me." But how is it possible that a similar thing is wrong with everyone? Logically this just didn't make sense. It reminded me of Garrison Keillor's fictional town Lake Wobegon "where all of the women are strong—and all of the children are above average." Isn't it more possible that something is wrong with the measurement tool?

Let's Hear It from the Ladies

That's how my excitement with the study started. The MRS study was an attempt to provide a new measurement tool and then create a conversation around it with this book, both to normalize female sexual behavior in midlife and to find patterns that might help us all understand what works and what doesn't. Selfishly, I wanted to feel better myself, and I wanted someone to tell me exactly how to do it. How lucky, honored, and humbled I am to be able to have this completely unfiltered and incredibly vulnerable information handed to me on a plate with the complete trust of the participants.

The study was designed as a survey which was sent by email to thousands of women ages 40–65 both in my own practice and also through my patients to other contacts. I have no idea how many people were exposed to the survey since it was shared through social media, email, and other channels. What I do know is that 1,013 women ages 40–65 completed the survey in the required timeframe. Another 600 or so completed it too late, and their responses were not included.

The final question on the survey asked if the respondent would be willing to be interviewed by me for this book. From the approximately 200 women who agreed to be interviewed, my research team looked for those women most likely to represent the angels of my prior experience: These were survey respondents who seemed to have figured out the secrets to a vibrant, spiritually connected sex life. This group was the mysterious sexually woke, and I could hardly wait to meet them!

My hope was that I could study these women and find out what they had in common, and then share it with the rest of us. What happened next were several months of incredible conversations with some of the most amazing group of women I have ever met. From more than 60 hours of transcribed recorded interviews, I struggled to pare down their wisdom into that which could fit inside this book and keep the rest for another time. Each of my transcribed conversations could have been published exactly as-is, and I hated leaving any of it on the cutting room floor.

What's Normal?

Starting with cold, hard statistics, most of us really just want to know if we are normal. I'm not quite sure what normal means, but I will use it to describe statistically average or midline behaviors. Normal for sure doesn't always mean optimal. But it really feels good to know that if you are struggling, you are not alone. We are all struggling.

If you are like me and hate statistics, I hope you can bear with me as I do my best to make this as readable as possible. While the study included women ages 40–65, we found that the 45–65-year-old age group more accurately reflected the struggles of midlife, so the data focused on the 715 women in this smaller age group, most of whom identified themselves as either peri-menopausal or menopausal. Two-thirds of this group reported currently having regular menopausal symptoms, with the single most prevalent adverse symptom being a decrease in sex drive (51 percent). Weight gain, fatigue, insomnia, and vaginal dryness rounded out the top five complaints. At the risk of sounding pessimistic, it's worth noting that many of the older women surveyed had already finished having symptoms, and some were already being treated and were complaint-free. Taking that into account, unfortunately only about 10 percent of women pass through menopause without noticing.

Of the women experiencing symptoms, weight gain was the single most negatively experienced or most disliked symptom (84 percent), followed by fatigue, insomnia, and decreased sex drive. Mood swings, depression, night sweats, hot flashes, and vaginal dryness all followed close behind. Needless to say, these symptoms are nothing to laugh about because they can seriously impact our lives and the lives of those around us, creating untold suffering.

Six out of 10 women felt they weren't prepared for menopause. They pointed to the internet as the top resource to learn about menopause with their OB/GYN doctor and friends falling second and third. This particular question made me quite sad. As an OB/GYN physician focused on menopausal health, it's clear that many of my colleagues are not doing their jobs for women in our age group. Teenagers at least go to a few puberty classes, albeit generally insufficient, but we get next to nothing to explain *What is Happening to Me? Part II.*

Rosie shares a funny story about this:

> So my mother never had the birds-and-the-bees talk with me. When I was pregnant, her only advice was, 'When I had you and your brother, I remember going to the hospital, and they gave me a pill. The next day I had a baby.' I was thinking to myself, 'Okay, so that was not helpful at all.' Then her story with menopause was the exact same thing. It involved a doctor, a pill, and then everything was perfect. My mother's recollection is she went to the doctor when she was 50, and he said, 'It's time to stop having a period.' He gave her a pill, and then that was it. Everything was sunshine and rainbows. I think our mothers remember things with a few gaps.

If you are a woman aged 40–55 and you are not asked a lot of questions about where you fall in the menopause spectrum when seeing your doctor and are not given some really useful information at your annual gynecologic exam, I suggest you find another provider. If you are forced to go to the internet for information, you become responsible to sift through mountains of garbage to find one pearl of wisdom. That's hard to do in a system meticulously set up to make you feel unworthy and entice you to buy something. It's a minefield.

Friends are really great to share what they've gone through, to provide empathy and hopefully a sense of normalcy, but they also can generalize their own symptoms and treatments to what is a very unique experience, which may leave you feeling even worse. Clearly this survey question about menopause resources confirmed what I already knew, which is that a huge information gap exists surrounding what to expect and how to manage one of the biggest transitions we face as women.

Despite the fact that nearly 7 out of 10 women currently or previously used hormones, most of them said they lacked knowledge about hormone options, risks, and benefits. This also speaks to the lack of education offered by many health care providers, assuming someone prescribed all these products. The old paternalistic style of "take this pill, honey, and you'll feel better," or worse, "take this handful of pills and creams that you can buy from my pharmacy right next door," negates our freedom of choice. Each of us has the right to choose what is best for us, and we should do so only after assessing the pros and cons of each option.

Let's Talk about Sex

Now for the exciting part that you have all been waiting for (or at least I was!). Just over three-fourths of women surveyed were sexually active with a partner. Of those who were not, nearly 9 of 10 wanted to be. For the active group, only half engaged in sex at least once a week. Thirty percent had sex once every two to four weeks, and 20 percent had sex less than once a month. Only 6 in 10 always or usually had an orgasm. I know that's a lot of numbers to swallow, so let's take a breather together and think this through.

First of all, what does "sexually active" mean? In the study we defined it as *intimate physical sexual contact* since vaginal intercourse certainly wasn't the only thing people were doing. Throughout this book whenever I mention sex, think of this broader definition. Keeping that definition in mind, since 90 percent of women in the study were married or in a relationship, that means more than 13 percent of women were not sexually active at all with their partner (remember, only 76 percent were sexually active). That's a tremendous number of sexless marriages or relationships. Put this way, if you know 10 women ages 45–65 in a relationship, one or more is not having sex at all, and more than two of them are having sex less than once a month. And if only 6 in 10 of those

If this sample represents what is going on with women across the Western world and possibly beyond, that's an awful lot of women not experiencing the joy of sex with a partner. Why isn't anyone talking about this?

who are sexually active always or usually have an orgasm, almost half always or usually do not. Bummer.

None of this was unexpected really after having heard it so frequently from patients in the office and living though it myself, but somehow seeing it on paper still surprised me a little. If this sample represents what is going on with women across the Western world and possibly beyond, that's an awful lot of women not experiencing the joy of sex with a partner. Having been one of them for most of my life, my heart sinks a little looking at those numbers. Why isn't anyone talking about this? To sum it up with another really telling statistic, two-thirds of women say they wish their sex life was different, and I don't think they wish it was worse. As I read this the first time, I thought, "Seriously, we need to make T-shirts or something and start a revolution. Why isn't everyone talking about this?"

A really interesting fact is that only 60 percent of respondents engaged in self-stimulation. I was surprised about that one; I thought everyone masturbated. It's also possible that in Texas it's not ladylike to admit it, even on an anonymous survey. Interestingly, nearly nine-tenths of those who self-stimulate always or usually have an orgasm. That's 50 percent more orgasms than with a partner. Clearly most of us know what turns us on, but apparently many of us are not communicating that to our partner, or something about the relationship is standing between us and an orgasm: embarrassment, fear of disapproval, shame, or resentment, among other possible reasons.

This is something I understand really well from personal experience. Since I was a small child, I could make myself have an orgasm easily and just about anywhere. I even got so good at it that I could make myself orgasm under the table with no hands in public with no one noticing. But with partners, it was not always so easy. If the only goal of sex was to have an orgasm, I could definitely handle that by myself and with much less work.

The fact that we are much more likely to have an orgasm alone than with our partner really speaks to the degree of relationship disconnection I've heard about so often for 20 years and have lived with myself. Sophie describes:

 In the last few years of my first marriage, I don't think I ever had an orgasm except alone. I just wasn't willing to be that vulnerable anymore. Years of building resentment had just shut that down. Orgasm for me became more about stress relief than anything to do with connection or relationship. When I needed to relax, sometimes I would masturbate. But the idea of having an orgasm with my ex-husband seemed like I was giving him too much. I wasn't going to do that anymore. I guess it was partly my way of telling him I was done. If I enjoyed sex, maybe our relationship had a chance, and subconsciously I knew it didn't. 🙶

One encouraging thing about this part of the study was the overwhelming desire to have sex by those who were not sexually active. With few exceptions, deep down, women want to have great sex. They may not want it the way they are getting it or with the person they are getting it with, but there seems to be a deep understanding that without it, something is missing.

I remember clearly when I was around age 40, a patient about my age came into my office and openly and confidently told me that she and her husband liked to try new things. She was concerned that she might have developed a vaginal infection from using her vibrator too much. She also had lots of questions about anal sex and whether it was safe. I remember her telling me that she missed having sex every day like they used to, and now with the kids in so many activities, they could only do it about three times a week. I tried to look unimpressed and nonchalant, but underneath I was full of envy and seriously wanted her life. I also realized I knew absolutely nothing about vibrators or anal sex and made up some useless advice about "as long as you enjoy it, it's fine." Of course, I warned not to go from anal to vaginal intercourse or she would get an infection. I made that up on the spot, but it seemed to make sense. I promise, we don't learn about this in medical school.

I thought about her for several days straight and even decided I was going to be more like her. Yep, I was going to go out and buy some sex toys and tell my then-husband I wanted to try new things and have sex three times a week. The desire for something different was so strong, but it turned out to be not nearly as strong as the resistance once I got home. Back in the reality of my non-communicative relationship and 100 excuses to be too busy, I just couldn't do it.

As it turns out, there is a big difference between wanting to do something and being willing to do it. Think about it. There are a lot of things that we want to do. So why is it that we don't do most of them? Being willing means letting go of a lot of things like old habits, excuses, resentment, and being right. And in this situation, there was no way in hell I was willing to do that. So nothing changed.

On to the next series of questions. It's probably not surprising that women report their sex drive to be highest in their 20s and that it falls over time. Sixty-one percent report that their sex drive was extremely strong or very strong in their 20s—only 48 percent before age 20—followed by 53 percent in their 30s, 34 percent in their 40s, 20 percent in their 50s, and 13 percent in their 60s. Although there are many factors that feed into libido, which are discussed in detail in Chapter Four, one that stands out to me while looking at these numbers is the desire to procreate. It's hard to argue with nature. Most of us don't want to get pregnant before age 20, even though our hormones are raging, and the average age for women in the United States to have their first child is currently 28.

In 2016 for the first time, there were more women in the United States having babies in their 30s than in their 20s, according to the CDC, which correlates with the finding that sex drive remains relatively high in the 30s and then starts to precipitously drop off. Why is this? When we are done having babies, our sex drive drops. At least that's my theory.

It's also not surprising that frequency of sexual activity drops with age. While more than 80 percent of the 45–49 and 50–54-year-old groups are sexually active, those numbers dropped to 66 percent and 59 percent in the 55–60 and 61–65-year-old groups, respectively. For those who were sexually active, the frequency of sex is remarkably similar across the 45–60 age group with about 50 percent having sex at least once a week and the other 50 percent less frequently. Only the 61–65 group has sex less frequently, with only one-third having sex at least once a week. While the study did not ask questions about partner health, my interviews confirmed that less-frequent sexual activity was often tied to erectile dysfunction and other male factor issues that become much more prevalent after 60.

One of the most interesting findings of this study was that only 4 in 10 women report being likely to achieve orgasm through vaginal intercourse. In fact, the two most likely ways to reliably achieve orgasm were with a vibrator or toy without a partner or manual stimulation without a partner. With a partner involved, the most reliable methods are pretty evenly matched and include a vibrator or toy, oral sex, and manual stimulation. Vaginal intercourse followed, and anal intercourse was dead last.

Stepping Outside the Box

This particular set of findings really highlights the need for us to step outside our boxes if we want to maximize our sexual experience, and our partners need to understand this. First, we clearly all need to have a good vibrator or two, and you don't need to go with a wig and dark glasses to a sex shop. In fact, you can order a personal massage device on Amazon.

My strong belief is that despite the fantasy of "cumming together," that phenomenon rarely happens, and the optimal sexual experience is a one-at-a-time situation. I personally can't concentrate on giving someone pleasure while fully immersing myself in my own pleasure. More often these days, I don't have vaginal intercourse at all or not as an endgame; rather I fully attend to what I am experiencing and then switch roles. I just don't think you can multi-task, and what's the rush? Plus in my experience, men generally fall asleep right after orgasm, but I can rally, so we take that into account with who goes first. Every couple is different, but there are also remarkable similarities.

Here's a sad statistic that I hope I can be part of changing. Almost 6 in 10 women say that their sex lives are worse at age 45–65 than they used to be, and only 7 percent say their sex lives are better. Obviously, what feels good changes with time. Half of women surveyed say they need more stimulation and time to achieve orgasm, while others say they could no longer tolerate certain activities due to dryness and pain or that some things that used to work just don't work anymore. Another bummer.

Despite that apparent lack of optimism, underlying these findings is hope. If 7 percent describe a better sex life, then it's possible. But we need to change things. We are not going to feel like we did when we were 25,

> Here's a sad statistic that I hope I can be part of changing. Almost 6 in 10 women say that their sex lives are worse at age 45–65 than they used to be, and only 7 percent say their sex lives are better.

and frankly who would want to? Both men and women need to adjust our sexual behaviors with age to align with the anatomic and physiologic changes that are inevitable. But importantly, what the sexually woke can teach us is that *we don't have to give up.*

When it comes to partnerships, only a little over half of women surveyed say they feel *very satisfied* with their relationship. On a positive note, many were actively working on improving their connection. Sadly, one-fourth say they want more out of the relationship but don't think it is possible, and 50 percent had been through a recent crisis. More than 1 in 10 women admit being unfaithful themselves, and 25 percent either know that their partner had been unfaithful or are suspicious. Half of women surveyed were either facing the serious illness or death of a parent or a serious illness themselves. Almost 10 percent were facing the serious illness or death of their partner. And we didn't even ask about children. Having three teens myself, I am guessing they would add to the suffering for many women. That's a lot of crisis. Without a doubt this is a potentially difficult time of life.

What's Sexy Now?

One really fascinating hypothesis prior to this study, at least to me, was that the things we find sexy in our fertile years are different than the things we find sexy in midlife. According to this hypothesis, when we are fertile, our primitive brain is looking for a mate who can provide for and take care of us. Subconsciously we are scanning for good DNA to keep our line alive. When we are no longer fertile and hopefully start to see sex as more of an opportunity for connection than procreation, the things we find sexy start to change.

> When we are no longer fertile and hopefully start to see sex as more of an opportunity for connection than procreation, the things we find sexy start to change.

Several questions were designed to dig into this, and the results were pretty much as expected. Women 45–65 said that many things are *more important* for sexual attraction now when compared to their 20s. These topped out with quality time, respectfulness, active listening, thoughtfulness, self-awareness, loyalty, and attentiveness. On the flip side, women 45–65 said that many things were *less important* for sexual attraction than when they were in their 20s, topping out with youthfulness, physical strength, receiving gifts, and physical attractiveness.

With these findings as the backdrop, I could give some advice to our partners having the typical "midlife crisis." There's no need to buy a red Ferrari, give expensive gifts, dye your hair, and attempt to look younger to be sexy to your 45–65-year-old female mate. Spend time with her, pay attention, listen, and be thoughtful about what she needs. That's red-hot sexy. Vanessa's perspective illustrates this eloquently, observing:

> As we get older, the quality I love the most about my husband is a kind heart. He listens to me, and I feel valued by him. That is really attractive and sexy to me now.

In another interview, Christina told me all about her second husband in deeply loving terms but never once mentioned his age, appearance, or career. What she did say is:

> I want someone who is going to listen to me ... to come up with ideas to help me accomplish the things I want to accomplish, and I will do the same for him. That's sexy. Or someone who says, 'You know what? You didn't get much sleep last night. Why don't I order dinner instead of you cooking tonight?' Somebody who wants to see you as valuable, that your opinions are valuable, your goals are valuable, you getting rest is valuable. Yes, I want to be valuable in that way. But you know what? When I was 20, I just wanted to be hot.

Further illustrating this, the great majority of women who had an affair or left their unhappy marriages for another partner did not do so while attempting to find a way out. Usually they connected accidentally with someone who really saw who they were, listened intently, and made them feel special and wanted.

Valerie described drifting further and further away from her husband who seemed disinterested in her when she was about 50. Occasionally she would go to a cafe just to be around people and began striking up a conversation with a man who also went there alone. After meeting a few times by accident, they began meeting on purpose. They would talk for hours. He laughed at her jokes and thought she was wonderful. Valerie started meeting him every day. Pretty quickly, sexual tension began to build. She realized how easy it would be to fall in love and have an affair. Instead, she confronted her husband, and they were able to find a counselor to get them back on track before things became irretrievable. When telling me this story, Valerie never mentioned what this man looked like, what his profession was, how old he was, or how much money he had. He didn't buy her gifts or make her promises. She fell in love with his attention to her.

A similar thing actually happened to me. When I was 46 and "happily married" to my first husband, I met a man at a triathlon race who was a fellow competitor much more experienced than me. I was blown away by the way he listened to me and how he seemed really in touch with and concerned about what I was feeling. He noticed that I was nervous even though I pretended not to be, and he asked me what I was scared of, which seemed like such an unusual question. In my entire marriage, I had never been asked something so deep and vulnerable. In fact, I was scared of the wind, so we talked about how wind was just wind for a while and about letting things be as they are.

We didn't see each other during the race, but he sent me a text afterward, which simply asked, "So??" Again, this seemed like such a beautiful and unusual question. Someone wanted to know about me, was curious about what I thought and interested in what I experienced. After the race, we returned to our separate lives in different cities but kept in touch and have remained friends. Through that single encounter, I realized there was a whole world of deeply vulnerable connection out there that I wanted but didn't have.

A few weeks later, I decided to leave my then-husband. I wanted to be with someone who looked at me and thought I was interesting and paid attention to my emotions—asked me how I was feeling—what I needed. Someone who saw me. Despite the terrific guilt and shame of knowing I was breaking up my "happy family," something beyond myself pulled me like a magnet, knowing that I was dying in that environment—or maybe more accurately could not be born—and that I needed to pursue a life of love and connection. When I wrote the list in my head (and later on paper) of the dream partner I wanted, it didn't say anything about appearance, income, status, profession, type of car, or even gender.

I wanted someone who would listen and laugh and make love to me passionately, who shared my spiritual understanding and wanted to live a life of service, personal growth, and loving with an undefended heart.

Those who want to hold onto their female partners would be well served to know this, and we women would be well served to tell them.

Comfortable in Your Own Skin

Weight and other age-related changes came up over and over again, both in my practice and in this study, as the No. 1 factor causing dissatisfaction. In fact, two-thirds of women surveyed said their weight was a significant problem. Fewer than 20 percent said their weight has stayed the same, and a resounding 86 percent perceived their metabolism has decreased in the past five years and that it was easier to gain weight. Almost half of participants said they worry about age-related body changes, and only 5 percent said they are totally fine with the changes of aging.

I can attest to the fact that weight increase in our 40s and 50s is a major bummer. Those who claim that decreasing metabolism around menopause is a myth have obviously never been a menopausal woman. As an athletic person, I have always been able to achieve the weight I wanted simply by changing my exercise routine for a week or two and maybe skipping dinner for a few days. It was easy to lose 10 pounds in a month. These days, staying slim is a daily battle. I can gain 10 pounds in a week on vacation, but it takes 6 months to get it off (at least I hope so; I still have eight pounds to go).

The above numbers illustrate the obvious. Our culture clearly does not embrace aging, and the way you feel about your physical appearance plays mightily into your sense of self-worth, which is highly correlated with libido. If you don't feel good about yourself, you don't want to be seen naked and vulnerable to a possibly critical eye, even if it's your own. Glenn Close was quoted in *The Guardian* saying, "It's one of these ironies I suppose, that we sometimes start feeling comfortable in our own skin only late in our lives, but hopefully with enough time to benefit from it." Being comfortable in our own skin and loving ourselves as we are is one of the single most important factors affecting libido.

The Spiritual Side of the Sexually Woke

The last group of questions in the MRS study centered around spiritual life. More than 80 percent of women described their spiritual life as important. More than one-third said they'd been seeking more spiritual guidance recently. Specifically, we didn't mention religion, and spirituality meant different things to different people. Interestingly just like me, 6 in 10 women said they had experienced some form of "midlife crisis" or midlife transformation.

To further flush out the sexually woke, my research team isolated three questions to which positive responses seemed to represent the sexually woke mentality:

1. **Sexual:** *"My sex life has become richer and fuller over time."*
2. **Connection:** *"We are generally really connected."*
3. **Spiritual:** *"My spiritual life is very important to me."*

When analyzing the data based on the answers to those questions, we found that the study showed that a shared spiritual practice was related to having a richer and more connected sex life. We also found that women who responded positively to these questions were significantly more likely to have a higher overall sense of well-being. While this might not be entirely surprising, it's worth spelling out that having a rich and connected sex life along with a vibrant spiritual life is associated with well-being or happiness. A spiritual life sometimes meant going to church or painting, writing poetry, being in nature, fishing, or practicing meditation or yoga. Having both a rich sexual and spiritual life is associated with higher well-being scores than having just one or the other.

Whether the chicken or the egg came first is a good question. Do happy people connect more and have better sex? Does connection and great sex lead to happiness? My sense is that it's a combination of both, and one feeds the other in a virtuous cycle. Positive responders also were more likely to initiate sex, which we used as a marker for libido.

Surprisingly to me, positive responders to these questions were not more common in young age brackets. In light of the previous observation that libido and frequency of sex decrease with age, these data show that sex (think physical intimacy) can still be as rich and as connected—or more so—when we are 65 as compared to 45, despite being less frequent.

Sexual Satisfaction and Surgery

Patients ask me all the time if there is something that can be done surgically to improve their sexual satisfaction. At the risk of losing you by seeming to contradict my previous statements about loving ourselves as we are, it seems like the answer for some women may be yes. Hang in there with this if you are feeling pushback or resistance, because in my experience both can be true, and in fact they are for me. I hope you can stay with me in openness and curiosity, or skip to Chapter Two.

I was part of a landmark study published in the Aesthetic Surgery Journal in April 2016 that followed women who had undergone either labiaplasty (to change the way the labia minora appear externally) or vaginoplasty (to tighten the vagina for improvement in sexual sensation). The study showed a significant post-procedure increase in perceived body image and sexual satisfaction for both groups of patients who were followed for two years. While I am absolutely not advocating these procedures for widespread use, the results can be life changing for certain well-chosen patients. Based on a routine survey sent to post-operative patients in my own patient base, more than 9 of 10 patients who underwent either surgical vaginoplasty or labiaplasty said they had a noticeable improvement in sexual satisfaction after the surgery.

Interestingly, there is no anatomic reason why labiaplasty should alter sexual function, so why did patients in this study show a significant improvement in both perceived body image and sexual satisfaction? The answer is presumably because these women felt more confident about the way they looked, which is a primary driver of libido. Since we are talking about what's "normal," almost all different shapes and sizes of labia minora are normal, just like almost all shapes and sizes of breasts and noses are normal. All body parts fall on a bell curve (a curve shaped like an upside-down U with ends that taper out), and while most people fall closer to the middle, many people fall closer to the ends. Someone has to be the tallest in the class, and someone has to have the smallest hands or the longest toes. But telling someone they're normal doesn't always help, particularly when normal doesn't feel—or look—optimal.

Many women seek out labiaplasty because it pinches when they ride a bike, pulls when they have sex, pokes out of their swimsuit, or creates a bulge in yoga pants. That's super annoying, and making that annoyance go away can dramatically improve quality of life. I stopped counting but having done well over 400 labiaplasty procedures in the past 12 years, I honestly can't recall having a patient who wasn't happy with the outcome of the procedure.

In addition to surgery, there is considerable evidence that several non-invasive procedures can also positively affect female sexual function. Injecting your own platelet-rich plasma (PRP) into the clitoris and anterior vaginal wall shows great promise in improving blood flow and sensitivity to that incredibly important area. PRP has been used for years in other applications for healing and increasing blood flow, and I have personally seen great results with it and have had it done myself! Other in-office treatments using various energy sources (such as radiofrequency, laser, or sound wave technology) intentionally create microscopic tissue damage to the clitoris and vaginal tissue, which in turn accelerates the production of new blood vessels and collagen and can greatly improve orgasmic potential. That being said, we can make the vagina and clitoris as healthy as it was when you were 30, but the brain is still the most important sexual organ in our body by far.

> My own experience as a woman combined with the MRS study results leave no doubt that sexual satisfaction is highly correlated with body image. It's easy to say that all these body changes are normal, but again, normal doesn't always mean optimal.

My own experience as a woman combined with the MRS study results leave no doubt that sexual satisfaction is highly correlated with body image. It's easy to say that all these body changes are normal, but again, normal doesn't always mean optimal. After I gave birth to my twins at age 37, returned to my baseline weight, and jumped back on my exercise routine, it was totally "normal" that my skin didn't shrink like the rest of my body. My belly skin hung down like an extra appendage. I was slim and worked out every day, but this empty sack of skin had to be tucked into my girdle undies to keep it from falling out on my lap at an inopportune time. Normal? Yes. Optimal? No.

I will forever remember the day I was driving, glanced down, and saw that my belly skin had rolled over the top of my low-waist jeans and was sitting on my thighs. After I pulled over and stopped crying, I called a cosmetic surgeon friend and scheduled a consultation for the next day.

I had a mini-abdominoplasty, or mini-tummy tuck (staying below and saving the belly button) when the twins were about two years old, after trying absolutely everything else first.

My breasts were also put back where they used to be, and I said goodbye to what looked like socks with a nipple on the end. After breastfeeding three babies, it's also "normal" to have almost no breast tissue remaining and an abundance of redundant skin. Now 12 years later, I still couldn't be happier. During those flabby tummy and saggy boob years, I hated to be seen naked, avoided sex like the plague, could never find a swimsuit that fit or was flattering and hid under a cover-up at the pool. My daily life was absolutely affected, and I spent a good deal of extra time finding appropriate undergarments or even vacation spots.

I am a huge proponent of loving yourself exactly as you are and accepting aging gracefully, and cosmetic surgery is absolutely not a fix for self-hatred, depression, or a delusional relationship with aging. But I would be a hypocrite if I didn't tell you that sometimes it really improves quality of life, because it improved mine. I also color my hair, whiten my teeth, and use Botox and other skin products that reduce the appearance of fine lines.

After my divorce, I felt temporarily terrified to be seen naked. No man had seen me naked except by ex-husband (and even then, not often) for 18 years, and the old body was not quite the same. Here's how I got past that. I recommend to anyone to put all of your physical vulnerabilities out on the table before you get naked with a new partner. After I told him about the wrinkle in one of my breast implants, my fear of being seen from behind due to my saggy bottom, and my collection of odd scars, we were able to make a comedy of what might otherwise have been dreadful. Having got all that out in the open, I was completely comfortable walking around naked in broad daylight or making love in the daytime or with the lights on, and cosmetic surgery is partially responsible for that.

I completely understand and agree with the argument that the patriarchy and the media put these ideas in our heads, and we need to stop trying to live up to unrealistic ideals. But the bottom line is that I feel better. I live my life with more confidence and ease. So I stopped viewing my body as a way to make a political statement and just made myself more comfortable. That's okay for me. And it may or may not be for you. Cheers to both.

Feeling confident about the way you look is a balance you must find for yourself, and perhaps we should resist judging the decisions others make. First because we are each firmly in control of our own body. And also because those judgments often reflect fears that we carry about our own body image. If this information doesn't resonate with you and your own body, then by all means throw it away. I completely understand how highly charged it may be for some of us.

So now we know what's "normal," perhaps you have found yourself somewhere is these pages and can start feeling less alone. I promise you, there is nothing you could think or feel that hasn't been experienced by countless other women. That doesn't make us each less unique and miraculous, it just makes us more connected.

TWO

Sex and Our Three Brains

Modern neuroscience has clearly mapped three unique areas of the brain that influence behavior in different ways. When we are young and fertile, the primitive part of our brain that ensures survival of the species has a very loud voice. This part of the brain is responsible for extremely primitive (sometimes called "reptilian") aspects of behavior, including primal responses to threat. The primitive brain is programmed by the desire to survive and drives behaviors commonly described as fight/flight/freeze. Animals will attack, run away, or play dead. In human terms, think of behaviors when you are triggered and feel emotionally endangered. There's no predator chasing us, but our old brain still resorts to its old tricks. We fight, run away, or shut down and pretend to be invisible. Can you relate?

Brain No. 2, the limbic brain, is in charge of relatively modern mammalian traits such as motivation and emotion. Third and most recent in our evolution, the prefrontal cortex is tied to cognitive and social behavior. High in the forehead, the prefrontal cortex controls uniquely human attributes such as reason and thinking, as well as higher order functions such as compassion, empathy, and guilt. Each of us has all three parts present and operating in our brains. So your responses depend not only on what you've experienced in your own life but also by millions of years of evolutionary inheritance.

The Clenched Fist

Our reptilian brain is anatomically and functionally the lowest part of our brain and is responsible for instinctual type behaviors. It's the part of your brain that makes you do things really fast and without thinking to avoid perceived harm, generally with the goal of keeping you alive when it thinks there's no time for an internal debate. This is a great idea when your life is in danger but doesn't turn out so well when the threat is an imaginary or an emotional one, and often leads to harmful reactive behavior.

The limbic brain is anatomically in the middle and responsible for motivation and emotion but lacks self-control. Popular psychology describes the "limbic highjack" that involves throwing a fit, having an anger outburst, or otherwise overreacting and then feeling bad about it once the prefrontal cortex comes back online.

Psychiatrist and neuroscientist Dr. Dan Siegel created a famous model of the brain as a clenched fist with the thumb tucked inside. (Dr. Siegel has a great video describing this on drdansiegel.com). In this model, the integrated or well-functioning brain has all three areas of the brain interconnected, importantly with the fingers representing the prefrontal cortex, connected to and holding the thumb, representing the limbic brain, in firm but gentle control. The reptilian brain is the base of your hand. If you extend your fingers, you can illustrate what happens when you "flip your lid." The prefrontal cortex is no longer in connection with the limbic brain, and your emotions are unchecked and can act without parental control. When you calm down and the fist returns to its original position, you're able to think through and create reason around your behaviors. That's about the time that I am apologizing profusely and feeling horribly guilty about acting in a childish or unevolved way.

> **Trying to thrive with a survival-programmed brain can be problematic and requires a good deal of self-compassion and self-awareness. That old brain keeps getting in the way of our peace and happiness.**

The human brain has evolved considerably since reptilian times, and if we can stay around long enough, who knows what the next phase of evolution will bring. There is considerable evidence that humans have even evolved in recorded history and that we are slowly becoming less violent and more peaceful. In *The Better Angels of our Nature*, Steven Pinker provides optimistic evidence that despite what we see on the news, we are living in the most peaceful time in humanity's existence. Most of our brain is still old and programmed specifically to survive. But at least in some parts of the world, we are able to have the space and freedom to consider how to thrive, not just survive. Trying to thrive with a survival-programmed brain can be problematic and requires a good deal of self-compassion and self-awareness. That old brain keeps getting in the way of our peace and happiness.

The mere fact that I've devoted a good part of my life to helping women have more fulfilling sex lives speaks to this fortunate position. When survival is pretty much taken care of, and you are more worried about having too much to eat than too little, you can start to think about how to be happy—how to thrive. If you're wondering what all this has to do with sex, I'll try to connect the dots for you.

Connecting the Dots

I remember clearly the primary driving force in my mid-20s to early-30s was to get married and have babies. My friends were all on the same mission. In retrospect, this was much more of a compulsion than a choice. I simply understood at a very deep genetic level that this needed to happen, and I set about constructing the conditions to make it possible. As it turns out, the person I was dating in my late-20s became the focus of that attention for biological survival. Statistically speaking, whoever you are dating in your mid- to late-20s will most likely end up being the person you marry.

Looking back, it's clear to me that very little of this had to do with free will, and almost all of it had to do with a subconscious biological drive to settle down and procreate. For me, as perhaps for most humans, marriage and childbearing was less of a choice and more of a compulsion brought about by hundreds of thousands of years of evolutionary conditioning. The icing on the cake is your own life's cultural conditioning.

In our culture, most women 25 or older start thinking they need to be married. In many other cultures, the age is much younger. Whoever you're dating is assessed through that lens. God forbid if you are 30 or older and dating. Look out! Whoever that guy or girl is will very likely turn out to be your spouse simply by the conditioning of our biology.

My first husband and I started dating when I was 28, so that radar was already on full alert. I feel sorry for anyone I might have started dating at age 28 because for sure he would have ended up being the victim of my obsessive need to be married. Granted, the "victim" had equal responsibility and shared the same delusional mentality, so I can only take 50 percent of the responsibility. But what happened, which is what happens with many people in Western culture, is that the person I was dating in my late-20s became my husband and the father of my children. Robin describes a similar experience:

> Looking back, I can see that each of us had a small sliver of wisdom because we didn't get married until five years after we met. Clearly there was some underlying understanding that this was not the right thing to do, but neither of us had the wisdom to own it. I do actually recall him saying it out loud once or twice. We were at an Astros baseball game maybe two years into dating, and somehow an excited fan leaned too far over the mid-outfield wall to try to catch a fly ball and fell about 20 feet onto the field. I immediately gasped and waited to see if he would move, and luckily he was not seriously injured. His girlfriend leaned frantically over the wall, waving her arms and screaming to check on his well-being but was unable to get to him. I turned to my beau and said romantically, 'I would have jumped over that wall for you.' He was silent.
>
> About a month later, during one of our periodic breakups, he recalled the incident and said, 'The thing is, I've been thinking a lot about that night, and I wouldn't have jumped over the wall for you. You are not the person I am meant to be with.'
>
> Although I knew he was right, I was absolutely heartbroken, felt a rush of childhood fears of being unlovable wash over me like a tidal wave and saw my fertility slowly slipping away. That was one of several breakups that ended when one of us had too much to drink and showed up at the other's house at 2 a.m. He actually even moved to another country for work. But we both missed the safety of being in a relationship so much that we conveniently forgot about our earlier revelation and decided to get engaged.

This was no love at first sight or soul mate true connection; it was a business arrangement based on our compatibility of intellect and moneymaking potential, as well as our age and a basic understanding that we could conform to societal norms and have the outward appearance of success.

Many other women shared similar stories. Alison describes a variation on this recurring theme:

It wasn't necessarily conscious, but part of it was because my friends were getting married. I remember those times when you're going to weddings every week and thinking, 'I've got to get married!' I'd been with him for two years and it was like, it's time. I felt like I was on a conveyor belt. We were just going along. We're going to get married. Then we had two kids because that's what you do. Marrying my first husband was for a totally different reason than my second. In my second marriage, we were both over 40, done with kids, and we are just really compatible. We love each other's company. I really love this person. I chose him, and he chose me. It's free will.

Partners and Psychology

Make no mistake. All types of psychological needs are met when you pick your partner. Mine was a deep need for security and stability after a completely insecure and unstable childhood. I also had a need to appear perfect and to fit in with the privileged group after having grown up suffering with having neither. So I found someone who I thought would heal those childhood wounds instead of bringing them into awareness and healing them myself.

In a similar way, Caitlin comments:

As far as his needs, after being badly bullied as a child, I think he was obsessed with power and social status. I was an executive, and he was too. He loved money, and we would have plenty of it. I was highly intelligent, pretty, and good in bed. Good breeding material. Most importantly, I agreed to marry him. Having previously been turned down by his first choice, he probably also felt like he was running out of time. All of this was out of awareness, of course, but looking back, it was clearly weighed by both of our subconscious minds and fueled by the primitive desire to settle down and procreate. 🙶

It's amazing how many red flags intelligent people can ignore when being driven by these instincts. We often settle because the other option seems too scary and may lead to our genes not being passed on. This is the realm of animals, not evolved humans. Animals are drawn by instinct and compulsion to procreate with no higher thought or true freedom in decision-making. I believe that humans have a higher calling if we listen for it.

Subconscious Patterns

Some men want to marry their mother while others rebel and marry the opposite. Women are often looking for a partner to mimic their "perfect" father or replace an abusive dad with another abuser, having been conditioned to believe this is what they deserve. There are as many versions of these subconscious patterns as there are humans with brains.

Many books have been written on the psychology of subconscious attraction. The bottom line stands firm and true: when a partner is chosen to heal wounds, it rarely ends well. We are looking for the missing piece to make us whole because we don't feel whole. I would speculate that most humans who marry and have children are operating, at least in part, from the same basic level. Some get lucky with their choice and find their true soul mate or become deeply connected later through lots of hard work, but the odds are low. While 50 percent of marriages end in divorce, a significant number of couples that stay married aren't happy. So a successful marriage or committed partnership becomes a long shot, at best, unless we go into it with our eyes wide open—or learn to open them later once we've suffered enough.

So there we are in our mid-20s to mid-30s operating with our primary driving forces being subconscious and coming from the primitive parts of the brain that seek desperately to survive, reproduce, and heal childhood wounds. This is not to say you cannot fall in love, have joy, and experience genuine happiness during these times—of course you can.

I recall having deep feelings of love for my first husband in those early years, but it was not the free type of love that can be experienced once I stepped outside the compulsion for reproduction and fitting in; it was always in the shadow of the need to keep this species moving forward and to have a sense of conforming to societal norms. I remember an intense sense of relief, of having "made it," to finally fit in and belong to the group of "normals." I was accepted into the Catholic Church, dutifully learned all the songs, prayers, and subtle body movements to look like I fit in: right knee genuflect, stand and kneel on cue, left hand over right to take communion, and absolutely do not drop the wafer. I did as I was told without asking questions. Belonging was more important than anything, even following a system that inherently did not satisfy my spiritual curiosity. All of my friends were getting married. We went to a wedding at least once a month, and baby showers were already starting on alternate weekends.

I've sat and cried countless times with women in their 30s and 40s who sense such an intense pain of not belonging, feeling abnormal, being disconnected, or looked down on by society simply because they hadn't conformed to the societal expectation of marriage and childbearing. Make no mistake. This drive is unbelievably strong, and the risk of not conforming can literally feel life-threatening. After I had that ring on my finger, I breathed a huge sigh of relief. I was not going to be one of those "abnormals." I belonged. Box checked. Now on to the next box.

THREE

Where Did My Libido Go?

When it comes to libido or sex drive, my personal experience, combined with that of thousands of patients, indicates periods of time marked by lots of willing sexual activity: dating years, early-marriage years and the baby-making years. Biology is driving us to attract a mate and procreate. So sex is often frequent, easy and rarely an issue of discontent for either party. Even during pregnancy, some women experience an increase in sex drive, driven by high levels of estrogen. And it goes without saying that puberty, with the onset of fertility, is marked by a high and often difficult-to-control interest in sex. It's hard to argue with biology.

From Procreation to Survival

After we meet our "perfect" mate, society and evolutionary programming usually tell us that it's time to start a family. I have personally experienced and heard stories from thousands of women recounting what happens next. Five or 10 years—possibly more—are blurred with exhaustion, coupled with ecstatic memories of early birthday parties and amazing feats performed by babies and toddlers, such as rolling over and saying their first words. Very little of that time has anything to do with a partner. The focus during those early childhood years is often almost entirely on the kids. Your partner may become a facilitator for the project of raising children rather than a three-dimensional person with a life and dreams of their own. The identity of a young parent can become entirely entwined with that of the children.

We lose ourselves. We often have no relationship with our partner outside of that shared with the children. It's no wonder that lovemaking and genuine connection, mindful listening, and careful, attentive conversation often go out the window. The two independent, self-reliant people who could engage in such behaviors have ceased to exist, or perhaps they never even got the chance to exist. Without an exceptionally unusual amount of self-reflection, self-awareness, and just plain work, this story repeats itself in many relationships.

Having small children is a frequent and legitimate excuse for not having sex. I vaguely remember having three children under the age of two years old. Without pictures to remind me that I was there, I would have remembered very little. Thankfully, the gift of digital photography has allowed me to revisit those times frequently and fondly. Getting married at age 33, I had difficulty getting pregnant and suffered several miscarriages before my son was born after a very complicated pregnancy at age 35. Thinking that another pregnancy would be difficult, we started trying for another child again right away using fertility treatments, and I became pregnant with twins before my son celebrated his first birthday.

So there I was at 37, with two premature newborns and a 19-month-old toddler. I also owned an incredibly successful and booming new business that was pulling me to work more than 80 hours a week. Needless to say, there were plenty of legitimate reasons not to think about sex. First and foremost, I'd had my tubes tied and had no desire to get pregnant. My primitive brain was telling me there was no further need to have intercourse. I was done having children. I was breastfeeding, and the accompanying low-estrogen state caused a temporary menopause-like vaginal dryness and decrease in blood flow to the clitoris. My breasts hurt. I was exhausted. I had three babies. I worked way more than full-time, including frequent 36-hour obstetrical night-call shifts.

This equation prioritized sexual activity somewhere below unloading the dishwasher and washing the car. It wasn't that I didn't care for my husband. In fact, I remember telling him my lack of sexual desire wasn't anything about him, rather I simply didn't want to have sex with anybody. If George Clooney had walked into the room naked proclaiming that he wanted me, I would have sent him home. Sex just fell off my list of things that were important. My sexual being went into hibernation.

Life moved from the biological desire for procreation to the biological need to survive so I could keep my babies alive. Winston Churchill was said to have described the history of humanity as "one more damn thing after another." This is how sex was to me: one more damn thing to do.

Unlike most things, sex was something I could avoid. Low-priority items on the list were pushed to the next day, and then the next. Life was a constant battle of putting out fires. Unfortunately, tending to my marriage was labeled as a low priority. Not uncommonly, once we have the security of thinking a certain part of our life is safe and does not need attention, we ignore it until it either starts screaming, acting out for attention or just walks away. As Karen describes:

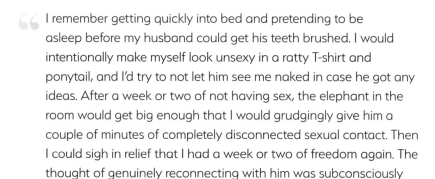

> I remember getting quickly into bed and pretending to be asleep before my husband could get his teeth brushed. I would intentionally make myself look unsexy in a ratty T-shirt and ponytail, and I'd try to not let him see me naked in case he got any ideas. After a week or two of not having sex, the elephant in the room would get big enough that I would grudgingly give him a couple of minutes of completely disconnected sexual contact. Then I could sigh in relief that I had a week or two of freedom again. The thought of genuinely reconnecting with him was subconsciously terrifying. It would be way too vulnerable.
>
> The fear of connecting prevented any real closeness since allowing him to rub my feet, give me a massage or snuggle with me on the couch might lead to sex. While I would have loved a free massage, I knew it was going to come with a price, so I avoided all intimacy like the plague. We became such strangers that the idea of sex with this stranger became not only scary, but also repulsive. Sometimes, I would grudgingly say yes and then try to push him away, but confused and frustrated, he would persist. It got so horrible I would tense up and cry.

Blurred Lines

In a marriage, our culture does not recognize this as sexual assault. Non-consensual or not-completely-consensual sex in marriage is rarely recognized as a reality, but it is much more common that you think. No one talks about it because it illustrates a deeply dysfunctional relationship and would, no doubt, lead to blame or allegations of revenge after the relationship ends in divorce. Non-consensual married sex may be one of the last flavors of sexual violence that women speak up and say "me too" about.

So many of us just put up with sex and live with it as a dreaded and constant reality. No doubt it's confusing for our partners, too. They hear, "Oh, is it that time again? I really just want to watch my TV show. But, I guess, go ahead if you really need to. Just make it quick." Hmmm. Does that mean yes or no? As a woman, I recognize this person does not want to have sex but is communicating in a passive voice and from a place of victimhood. She most certainly is not saying yes. For women, without a "whole body yes," sex should not continue because if it does, *it feels non-consensual.*

Back to Hmmm. What the man heard was "Go ahead." Both parties are responsible for unclear communication, and the result is disastrous. Without studying and practicing new ways of clear communication and some serious counseling, anger and resentment can grow to unbearable levels and something will inevitably crack.

Unraveling

Eventually, children are old enough to not need their parents every moment of the day. Then what? Mom and Dad (or partner and partner) are suddenly faced with seemingly endless swaths of time because the children don't need them constantly, and they're forced to look at each other and have a conversation. More often than not, these two people don't know each other anymore. They joined together in marriage or partnership through a likely immature love fueled by some subconscious biological compulsion, followed by years of distraction with young children needing their complete attention. Now they are two strangers. The choice at this point is either to pile on more delusion or to wake up. Since we already know that half of marriages in the United States end in divorce, and many of those who stay married are admittedly deeply unhappy, the most common strategy is clear.

The average time to divorce after the first marriage in the United States is eight years. Not surprisingly, that's just about the same amount of time it takes to get pregnant, have babies and nurture their growth to an age that doesn't require your constant attention. It's the same number of years that it takes to come full circle, finally look at each other in the eye and realize you're living with a stranger—possibly one you don't even like.

When my son was around three years old, I was in bed on a Sunday morning and heard the toilet flush. Anyone with children understands what a momentous occasion that is. About a year earlier, he turned on the television in the living room by himself to be entertained by "Baby Einstein" while we "slept in" (think 7 a.m.). However, flushing the toilet indicated a whole new level of independence. If he could entertain himself and go to the bathroom by himself, approximately half of my previously occupied time had now opened up. Of course, I had twins 19 months behind him who also had to go through a similar transition, but as predicted, they followed the same growth path. Sooner or later, they didn't need me every minute.

While the gradual and growing independence of my children slowly loosened their grip on my responsibilities and time, it took until they were in second or third grade before there weren't still plenty of excuses to divert all of my attention toward them. Once they were seven or eight years old, sleeping all night, making their own breakfast, dressing themselves, going to the bathroom by themselves, and packing their own bags for vacation, it was much harder to avoid being married. Not surprisingly, this eight-years-into-parenthood timeframe is when many relationships fall apart or, at the least, need a lot of compassionate attention. Certainly, this is what happened for me, and it's corroborated by national statistics.

The Elephant in the Room

Piling on more delusion can come in many forms. Not talking about our feelings, pretending things are okay, starting solitary hobbies that seclude us, traveling more for work, having affairs or just giving up are all common tactics that avoid the elephant in the room. I became an Ironman triathlete, participated in several races a year and started traveling regularly to Africa for mission work when my kids were eight and 10. Not coincidentally, my then-husband started traveling much more for work. These are socially acceptable and even laudable behaviors, but there is absolutely no doubt that we were creating very clever plans to avoid each other, to be too tired for sex or to listen openly and to connect.

Luckily, my line of work provided ample opportunities to share stories with patients and colleagues that made me feel normal. I was in my late-30s and early-40s, sharing lighthearted stories with patients that made us giggle secretly to mask our silent shame. "Sex for me is similar to what going to the gym is like for my husband," I would declare. "I love going to the gym, but he hates it. When he finally goes to the gym, he says he'll be going back three times a week, and it never happens. It's just not natural for him. He has no desire. It's just something he does once in a while because he thinks he has to."

I had another joke I made to cheer up patients who felt ashamed and alone in their lack of sexual desire. "If my husband had a disease that made his penis fall off, I would console him, but secretly I would be super-relieved because it would be one less thing to do." Everyone liked that one. They could relate.

Common Enemy Intimacy

The degree and apparent normalcy of such conversations is heartbreaking in retrospect. While my jokes had the effect of connecting with my patients and sharing true-life experiences that made us all feel better, the truth is that this was a pseudo-connection based on a shared shame and unspoken longing for something more. This was really a form of what author and research professor Brené Brown calls "common enemy intimacy," a substitute for genuine connection based on the common dislike of something or someone else. While I eventually got out and now live on the other side of that very sad space, I often wonder how many women are still trapped in a personal prison to which they hold the key, waiting for the courage to tell themselves they deserve something better.

A variation of this scenario happens for those suffering from infertility or pregnancy loss. Caitlin explains it this way:

> The first three years of my marriage were almost entirely absorbed by infertility, and it gave us something to focus on—or obsess about—that became our shared hobby. In that respect, we had things to do together—doctor's appointments, surgeries, grieving, counting days on the calendar—and something to talk about. It may have been the time that we were the closest. There was a reason to have sex and a reason for us to be together that we didn't have to think about.

This is another example of common enemy intimacy, that pseudo-connection that comes from aversion to the same thing. Luckily for Caitlin, she was eventually able to have two children after several miscarriages and surgeries. But many couples suffer much longer with less fortunate outcomes, and many marriages have ended due to the overwhelming emotional and financial stress of infertility. After losing the dream of a "normal family," a tidal wave of blame, resentment, and loss of emotional connection often crashes in.

The Crossroads

Like all things worth doing, waking up involves way more work than hiding in the dark. For sure, I didn't want to do that work during my first marriage, nor did my spouse. It involves self-reflection and accepting your partner and yourself exactly where you are now, combined with a vision of where you want to be as a couple. It requires a genuine curiosity and deep interest in what is best for each person and the partnership every day for the rest of your lives. That's no small feat. As with any crossroads, you have a choice.

Some of my patients, like me, took on multiple hobbies as distractions, spent less and less time with their mates, slowly drifted apart, and got divorced. Things were just too broken to be fixed.

One sadly funny memory that Carla shared occurred after a daylong intensive counseling session with her then-husband, which took place over a weekend. Having spent all day with them, the therapist said, "Usually at this point, I recommend that you go back to your hotel, get naked, and just lay on the bed together and see what happens. But for you two, don't do that. I'll see you in the morning." At the end of that weekend, her spouse confirmed what Carla already knew. Their relationship was over.

Many of my patients have stayed married and became progressively more unhappy, sometimes having affairs or engaging in other numbing behaviors with shopping, alcohol, pornography, or buying new cars or houses. They put off happiness for another time, until after the kids were grown, until after the scale showed 20 pounds less or until after (fill in the blank). Others, like me, found a new partner and a new playing field with an atmosphere in which to finally experiment with being authentically connected. A smaller number became genuinely reconnected with their long-term partner and found the passion that brought them together in the first place.

Anatomical Realities

In this overview of sexuality's life course, it's important to recognize the biological changes that menopause adds to the sexual conundrum. Anatomically and physiologically, decreasing estrogen and just plain aging cause potential problems for our libido. As we age, the vaginal lining becomes thinner, less elastic, and produces less moisture. Blood flow to the clitoris and vagina decreases, and the clitoris shrinks. Nerves responsible for pleasure become less prominent and less sensitive. Reaching orgasm can become difficult or seem impossible. Vulvar skin disorders like lichen sclerosis can cause the tissue to be even more fragile and painful to touch.

If an activity is going to hurt or at the least not be pleasurable, our bodies naturally will not be drawn to it. These factors make it unlikely to fully relax into the completely present and surrendered state necessary for true intimate connection. Luckily, this is not the case for every woman, and treatments exist for those who suffer with vaginal dryness and pain. It's no wonder decreasing libido is one of the most frequent complaints that brings patients to my office in the 40-plus age group.

Despite these anatomic realities, I still firmly believe the old saying that I learned in medical school: 90 percent of libido for men originates from below the waist, while 90 percent of libido for women originates from above the neck. These numbers are not likely the result of a rigorous study, but the point is well made.

As a broad generalization, sex drive for men seems to be much less affected by their emotional state, sense of intimacy, and desire for connection than for women. A pill that simply increases blood flow to the penis works wonders for male libido but has been shown to have very little effect for women. In other words, regardless of the anatomic and physiologic state of your female genitals, if your brain isn't into it, you won't want to have sex.

A recent study by University of Michigan psychology professor Sari van Anders showed that testosterone given to post-menopausal women increased the desire to masturbate but did not increase the desire to have sex with a partner. Even when we are aroused biologically, the desire to make love with a partner originates in a desire to be intimate and connected. Having an orgasm is something we can achieve easily on our own. Intimacy and connection are much more difficult. Alexa clarifies:

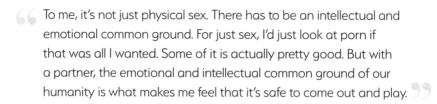

> To me, it's not just physical sex. There has to be an intellectual and emotional common ground. For just sex, I'd just look at porn if that was all I wanted. Some of it is actually pretty good. But with a partner, the emotional and intellectual common ground of our humanity is what makes me feel that it's safe to come out and play.

In another interview, Crystal jokes:

> We learned how to make our communication really clear. He will ask, 'Are you sleepy?' which is code for 'Do you want sex that's going to last 10 minutes or half an hour?' If I'm sleepy, I can say, 'Give me a second; let me go get the vibrator.' If he's tired, we can figure something out. 'I understand if you're tired, and I can make it quick. But I want you to participate because I can easily go in another room and have an orgasm. That's not the point. I want to connect with you.' We work together to find a middle ground.

Behind the Wheel of Libido

Libido for women is complicated, to say the least, and what drives it changes throughout our lives. In our teens, libido is driven by hormones and the biologic reality of our fertility, combined with the desire to be loved and accepted. As we get older, libido is driven by the desire to find and attract a mate and/or by the pre-programmed desire to procreate. But what drives the desire to have sex when we already have a mate, we are no longer fertile, and our genitals seem to be systematically shutting down? Clearly, it's not biology anymore. To find the answers, I had to get divorced, find true love, and experience deep authentic spiritual connection for the first time. I also had to ask more than 1,000 women for their perspectives and expand my search to include not only the scientific but also the spiritual world.

And I also had to come to an important realization: the last years of sexual life are deeply rooted in the first years. Ironically—and poignantly—we have to reconnect with and accept our childhood self to move forward with freedom. It can be harder than you imagine yet more liberating than you expect. For this reason, the next section of this book is about just that.

"Do not try to save
the whole world
or do anything grandiose.
Instead, create
a clearing
in the dense forest
of your life
and wait there
patiently,
until the song
that is your life
falls into your own cupped hands
and you recognize and greet it."

—*Martha Postlewaite*

PUTTING IT TOGETHER

FOUR

Sex and Early Experience

A s a parent of teenagers, I often wonder about the stories they will tell their spouses and psychologists about all the ways my parenting failed them. My parents screwed up. My parents' parents screwed up. I'm possibly the first generation that has finally learned how to parent perfectly and raise completely emotionally balanced adults who are open and ready for complex relationships and healthy sex, but I doubt it.

My sex education was pretty much a disaster. The great void that was left by my parents and teachers just not being willing or able to discuss the subject created an open playing field in which I was completely vulnerable to whatever outside input presented itself. The result was a bunch of pain and suffering that could have been avoided, and it created a view of sex that was certainly not based in love and compassion. Only by sheer luck did I not have an unintended pregnancy, contract a nasty STD, or get seriously hurt.

Determined not to make the same mistake with my kids, I've attempted to create a home environment where we can discuss anything and everything about sex and be completely open and unashamed, but this has not always been received quite how I hoped. When I try to start a conversation about sex, my kids typically roll their eyes and beg me to stop, insisting, "Mom, you are so embarrassing!" Apparently I am much more interested in sex than they are, but at the very least, they will be armed with an abundance of knowledge. We will see how that turns out.

The Impact of Lessons Learned

So much of how we think, believe, and behave as adults is impacted by lessons learned earlier in life. This may sound obvious, since growing up is a constant process of learning and applying those lessons to our understanding of the world. Learning how to drive a car, play the piano, or perform surgery, and then applying that knowledge is generally beneficial, assuming you have a good teacher.

As an OB/GYN resident, I had some of the best and worst surgeons as teachers, and both taught me equally important lessons. But learning in personal relationships is different, particularly in primary loving relationships. When the lessons are painful, an unconscious pattern of self-protective behavior can develop that does not apply to the current circumstances. The term "projection," loosely described, applies to the misapplication of a feeling or behavior that was learned in an earlier relationship to another person or relationship. Said another way, you can project your own feelings onto your partner, misunderstanding that they're feeling what you are actually feeling. In other instances, you project or transfer the feelings from an old relationship onto the current one. For example, if my first husband read the paper when I was talking to him, I might get overly sensitive when my current husband seems not to be paying attention to me.

From the day we are born, sexuality is a minefield of mostly really unhelpful pieces of information that are fed to us by our parents, church, schools, friends, doctors, music, art, photos, movies, and the media. Sex is everywhere, attached to confusing messages about what you should and shouldn't do, good and bad, right and wrong. This is one of my favorite hilarious-but-true quotes:

"Life in my small town of Lubbock, Texas taught me two things. One is that God loves you, and you are going to burn in hell. And the other is that sex is the most awful, filthy thing on earth and you should save it for the one you love."
—Butch Hancock

Our brain does its best to sort this information into a story that makes sense and combines it with our personal experience from early relationships. Of course, each of us constructs a different view of reality. We show up in our relationships with these views like an overstuffed suitcase. Your partner shows up with a completely different type of personal baggage. As my meditation teacher Vinny Ferraro often jokes, what could go wrong?

The Weight of Baggage

In my case, a lot went wrong. Before I completely throw my parents under the bus, I truly believe everyone does their best with the resources they have at the time. That doesn't absolve us of accountability or consequences for our actions, but it does release us from blame. Assuming you do the best with what you have, it is safe to say that sometimes your best is pretty crappy, and everyone else's best is equally crappy at times too.

In my mother's case, she was dealt a pretty bad hand, including strict, emotionally unavailable and unloving parents, emotional and social immaturity, debilitating shyness, a rigid Christian upbringing, and an unavailable, disconnected spouse. She married my father in her early-20s because it was the "right thing to do." My father regretted his proposal shortly after he made it but was too scared to cancel the wedding in case she went off the rails. Although the diagnosis was never officially made, my mother fits the description of Borderline Personality Disorder, which is marked by intense and changing moods, intense fear of abandonment, cycling love-hate relationships, and threats of self-harming behavior. No wonder he didn't want to call off the wedding. My father and our family lived in constant fear of one of her tantrums, and we revolved around her ever-changing moods.

One thing my mother loved was a baby. She was a doting caretaker to my sisters and me as newborns because we completely depended on her. We gave her a sense of purpose and the illusion that we would not abandon her, but once we started to walk and talk, everything changed. The two-year-old talking back and having tantrums of her own sent my mother into a tailspin. She was completely ill-equipped to handle this type of conflict and would retreat to her room where I imagine she eased her suffering by planning to have another baby. Somehow my mother manipulated my father into having five children, allowing her to enjoy at least five years of her life with the unwavering love of a newborn. I regret that I can't remember that first year of life with my mother; it was the one and only time we ever connected.

When it came to sexuality, my mother was completely shut down and terrified. She was so uncomfortable with anything to do with genitalia that she didn't ever say a word to me about puberty or periods. I was left to figure that out by myself. Unfortunately, my period started at age 11, and I spent two years making homemade pads out of tissues and safety-pinning them to my underwear. I lived in constant fear of an accident and feigned many days of illness to get out of going to school. When I was 13, a box of sanitary pads arrived on my bed with no explanation or discussion, and that pattern continued until I could use my allowance to buy them myself.

Unconsciously—my mother will never admit it and swears it was just fashion—she made herself and all of her daughters plain and inconspicuous, keeping our hair asexually short. Our clothing was conservative and as long as she could force it, was matching. I hated my short hair. I clearly remember wearing shorts and a T-shirt around age 8 and being mistaken for a boy, just when I was becoming terribly self-conscious about my chubby body and ugly hair. I was devastated. As soon as I was physically and mentally strong enough to flat out refuse to cut it, I grew my hair long and have had it long ever since. Haircuts are still hard for me,

> I think my mother's unconscious wish was to keep me safe from the sexual world that she perceived as dangerous. That plan backfired completely.

and both of my daughters have had long hair since it was able to grow as toddlers. The certainty that I was ugly stuck with me until I was late in my teens. I think my mother's unconscious wish was to keep me safe from the sexual world that she perceived as dangerous. That plan backfired completely.

My teenage years tell a tragic story of a very sad girl who would do just about anything to get someone to like and accept her. Combined with neglectful parents who were too busy with their own personal crises to set any boundaries or establish consequences, you can imagine how that unfolded. In retrospect, I suspect my mother was sexually abused. Her sister seemed similarly sexually repressed, and their father was a strange character indeed. My grandfather, a physician, was apparently completely disconnected from his wife, who I remember as being the meanest grandmother on earth. She thought that children should be seen and not heard. I was terrified of my grandmother and was relieved that she died when I was 10. She had seen me only three or four times in that 10-year period, and every visit was petrifying.

There was plenty of suffering in that family, and I imagine my mother did the best she could with her extremely immature and limited capacity. Although she was a math genius and earned a master's degree in statistics and early computer programming, my mother had the emotional intelligence of a small child. She was traumatized as a child, I am guessing and was emotionally stuck at that same age forever.

I share all of this not to gather sympathy or to pass the blame on to others, but simply to give an example of how things happen. I know many readers have similar stories. Despite my less than perfect upbringing, I am completely satisfied with where I am now and have nothing but gratitude and compassion for the people who helped get me here.

The Birds and the Bees: Shhh

The lack of sex education from parents of our generation was almost ubiquitous in the MRS study. Almost every patient describes getting nothing more than the required and terribly inadequate class at school, a pamphlet or book, or a very short, uncomfortable conversation about the birds and the bees that left out most of the important details. In fact, only one woman out of all of those interviewed, Daniella, described a fully open and ongoing conversation with her mother about puberty and sex. Daniella grew up in the 1960s and '70s with what she described as "Bohemian parents":

 They were like Beatniks and were very artsy. I was raised in a very close and very liberal family. Mom and Dad talked about sex. I always say communication was my parents' secret to successful relationships. I could talk to my parents and tell them anything. They'd ask me about drinking or drugs or anything like that. I could tell them the truth. They were very affectionate to each other and to me; I was cuddled and held a lot. I remember mom talking to me about sex at an early age, and I knew she would always be supportive with those kinds of issues.

When I was 16, mom took me to Planned Parenthood and made sure I was on the pill. I lost my virginity in 10th grade just as an experiment. It was passionate and felt great, but I knew nothing was going to come out of it. There was no guilt or shame or anything. I knew my parents went through sexual experiences and adventures, so I've always had openness about sex. I've always been kind of curious about what people do to pleasure themselves together and alone. Sex was always an important part of my relationships. I had a lot of sexual partners before I met my husband, and all of them were fun. I never had a bad experience. Since I've been married, sex has always been a part of our daily lives. At first, we had sex at least once a day, and at times it has been less than that, but we have always had a sexual connection of some sort every day when we are together. It is just part of who we are.

My husband and I have always been so in love with each other physically, even after 26 years of marriage. Sometimes I wear a bathrobe or whatever, but most of the time I am naked. I'm not hiding from him. I don't have the lights off or anything; it's just me. He loves me the way I am at 56, and I love him the way he is.

Many other women remembered their sex education, or lack of it. Let me share a few of those stories in case you can connect with them. Alison doesn't remember being taught anything directly about sex by her parents, although she clearly recalls learning that sex was healthy and fun:

My parents always had a healthy sexual relationship, and it was always out there. My dad was always chasing my mom. He'd come and hug her all the time, and they were very much in love. They didn't make it a secret that they were having sex. It was something very open. I have always known that sex was a really important part of relationships, and it's been something that I have been very comfortable with.

Kimberly, who married her childhood sweetheart as an 18-year-old virgin, recalled a completely different experience. She remembers:

> I grew up in a strict Baptist home. You don't talk about sex. You don't dance. You don't do this; you don't do that. We came from blue-collar working families. They weren't well-educated people. Nobody questioned getting married at 18. It's just what was expected. If you were lucky, you would finish high school, get married, and get a job to support your kids. Nobody ever thought of anything more. I had my first baby at 21 and then quit working since that was what people did. It was a different time.

Victoria also married her childhood sweetheart as an 18-year-old virgin. She describes coming from an "unhealthy family" with an alcoholic mother. Victoria was largely raised in foster homes:

> I did not have a good thought about sex. I thought sex was dirty. When I was 12, there was bad stuff going on with my mother around sex, with men coming over and the like. I was scared to death of sex. I didn't want to make myself attractive to men and was terrified when I got breasts that men would want me in that way.
>
> We married right out of high school, and we had to learn a lot of things by scratch. At first, sex to me was like a chore. I would do it just for him, and neither of us had a clue about anything but the basic way. My husband was very patient and kind, but I didn't even have a climax for years. On our wedding night, we didn't even have sex because he finished too soon. It was all really funny looking back on it. We were thrown into marriage with no clue of what to do.

Sadly, Crystal's first sexual experience was at age six when her stepfather molested her, a nightmare that continued until she was 13 years old:

> He abused my sister and me sexually, mostly touching, and not sexual intercourse, but still, it was bad. My first experience with sex was confusing. He threatened me not to tell anyone and said it was normal. I was just a child.

At age 13, Crystal told her mother and was sent to live with her father, but her mother denied that the molestation happened. Crystal recalls her father saying, "Sex is special; keep it to yourself," which gave her more self-confidence. She describes:

> I guess I went through a control thing thinking, 'It's mine. I'm going to keep it, and I can give it away if I want to.' I started being sexually active at age 17, but I was just exploring with guys. I was just trying to figure out what I liked and what I didn't like. I was never faithful to one boyfriend because I thought, 'This is mine. I can give it to whoever I want.'

It's easy to understand how Daniella and Alison's upbringings and early conditioning created an approach to sex that was free, healthy, and without guilt and shame, and how Victoria, Kimberly, and Crystal had to work hard to repair the damage done by caregivers who made sex seem taboo and unhealthy. Hopefully as parents, grandparents, and influencers, we can learn from our own parents' mistakes—remember, they did the best they could with their own conditioning—and help raise a generation of young women who are free of the baggage around sex that so many of us share from early childhood.

Like me and many others, Helen had a unique experience as a teenager that shaped her perception of sex:

> The only concern we had as teenagers back then, as I recall, was pregnancy. This was before AIDS, and nobody really had much of an idea about sexually transmitted diseases. Dad was a doctor, and he made sure I was on the pill when I needed to be. That was his entire contribution. There was no discussion about it. He just sent me along to his friend the gynecologist, and I was on the pill at age 14.
>
> Before that, I had gone to a mother-daughter evening at school, but there was no follow-up or discussion. When I had my first period, I was totally unprepared. I didn't know what was happening, and it was quite frightening. I told my mother, and she simply directed me to a cupboard that had supplies.

Helen's best friend and constant companion from age 13 to 17 was her childhood sweetheart Mark:

> I led a very sheltered life, but my older sisters had boyfriends, so I saw them coming and going. The girls at my high school talked about boys in terms of being objects of desire. I guess that's where most of my ideas about sex came from. I was very lucky that Mark and I had a very stable and mature relationship. We were best friends and kind of learned about sex together. It was a really healthy relationship. He was always with my family. My home was like a second home to him and his to me. We walked to school together and grew up together through those years, and it kept me safe through that period of my life. I expected that we would get married and be together forever, but at about 17, we just grew apart.
>
> I think our relationship was absolutely fundamental in laying the groundwork for my orientation to sex. Sex was a wonderful, enjoyable experience for me with him. For many decades after, that was the best sex of my life. I thought, 'That's it; it's over now. It's never going to be that good again.' We were young, fit, and didn't have any inhibitions or hang-ups that came into my life later on. As long as people are in a loving, stable, and monogamous relationship, it can be such a wonderful time to have sex when we are young. I've never been of the opinion that you need to wait until you get married.

Not surprisingly, sex and religion became entwined in less-than-healthy ways in many of our lives. When Helen got married in her mid-20s, she followed a religion that taught sex was only for procreation and should not be enjoyed. Consequently, she describes:

> All the young married couples were beset by guilt because no one could follow those rules. There was a huge amount of guilt around sex. It really destroyed people. Everyone was walking around pretending to be somebody they weren't. It was really destructive to people. After we had our two children, we became so disconnected that sex was just awful. It was just something I felt I had to do for him. I was married for 19 years when my husband

left me for a younger woman. He blamed me because I hadn't been fulfilling his sexual needs, so it was my fault.

With a different but equally confusing history around sex and religion, Rosie came from a strict Catholic family. She laughs about the mixed messages she received:

> I had a boyfriend when I was 15 and started to have all these amazing feelings for this person. All of a sudden, I was being told, 'Those feelings are okay, but you are not allowed to do anything with them unless you are married.' There was always this sense that when we were together it was really great, but it felt dangerous because it was pushing us toward doing something that morally we weren't supposed to do. We would have this really great feeling when we were close, then we would get scared and stop. It was like, 'That was really great, but that was something we weren't supposed to be doing.'
>
> The conversation my teachers had with us in health class was very, very clinical and did not make sex seem attractive at all. It was all about the pitfalls. You could get pregnant, you could get a disease, you could ruin your reputation and your family, and you could go to hell. But once you got married, it was a gift from God. I kept thinking it was so hilarious because I've got this gift—God was like the guy who kept giving and taking away. Here you are your whole life being told you're not supposed to have sex, and then all of a sudden you are married. And you're wondering, 'Am I doing this right? I don't know anything about sex. Are there things I should be doing better?' All these questions would bubble up.

Enter Stage Left: Charlene

In contrast to Daniella, most of what I learned about sex came from three sources: the 1973 pair of cartoon books titled *Where Did I Come From?* and *What's Happening to Me?* that were left on my bed without discussion, the secretly procured *The Joy of Sex*, and my friend Charlene.

I was always the youngest in my class, and at age 13, I met Charlene during our first year of high school. Almost a full year older than me, Charlene was tall, beautiful, worldly, and completely wild. In 1980,

Charlene had mastered the Farrah Fawcett hairdo with a center part and bangs winged toward the back. She knew how to hold and puff casually on a cigarette and reportedly had already had sex with a boy in the bushes behind the middle school. She knew dirty words I'd never heard, but I pretended to never be surprised. For two years we were inseparable; Charlene was my first true love. She was also the first person I ever had sex with. Playing around one day after a significant amount of alcohol, she decided to "pretend we are lesbians." As usual, I went along. The game only stopped when my bleeding and pain, which were both significant, scared us both.

Although I have never been able to reconnect with her as an adult and hear her side of the story, her bravado and out-of-control behavior must have been masking some deep pain that I never learned about. At the time, I thought Charlene was magical and would have done just about anything she suggested. I was a loyal and faithful wing-woman, always allowing her to take the spotlight and enjoying whatever remnants of attention and adoration came my way from being by her side. Being Charlene's best friend made me special, and I accepted my role as the less pretty one without hesitation. She made me feel like I was good enough, and although neither of my parents had ever told me that they loved me, I knew Charlene did.

For reasons I didn't question at the time, Charlene and I were rarely supervised outside of school. I don't recall having any rules, curfews, or consequences. We spent the weekends talking for hours on the phone and took the bus to the mall, roller skating, and the beach, where we would smoke cigarettes, drink a mixture of hard liquors stolen from our fathers' cabinets, and attract the attention of any number of similarly unsupervised boys. Most weekends, someone would have a party at whoever's house had no parents. I was way out of my league hanging out with a wild bunch of kids older than me, but I feigned confidence to be accepted in their super cool circles. At this point, my sexual experience included kissing a boy at the end of a middle school dance, my drunken game with Charlene, and giving myself what I later learned to be an orgasm by climbing a rope or a pole starting around age five.

The Other Big O

As an aside, I got really good at climbing ropes and poles as a child, and when I later read about what those sensations were that I was experiencing, that there was a name for them—orgasms—and that other people had them too, and particularly that you could have them with another person, I was flabbergasted. Few people know that about 10 percent of girls have orgasms well before puberty, as early as age two.

While little boys are known to play with themselves and have erections, they are not able to have an orgasm until puberty. Little girls, however, are sometimes able to have very satisfying orgasms surprisingly early on. One of my friend's daughters inherited this talent and began "squeezing her legs" around age three. For a while, she would do it almost daily wherever and whenever the mood struck her, including at restaurants, the park, and in her stroller. She would squeeze and straighten her crossed legs rhythmically until her face turned red and her eyes rolled back in her head, and then she would melt into a state of pure relaxation. Had I not experienced something similar, I would have wondered if she was having a seizure. Luckily, her mom and I were able to talk about it and teach her beautiful girl that it's perfectly fine and fun to squeeze your legs, but it's something you should do in the privacy of your room since it involves your "private parts." I haven't seen her squeeze her legs since she was four or five, but I'm pretty certain she has evolved her techniques as a 15-year-old teen who no doubt spends plenty of hours alone in her room with way more resources than I had at her age.

Fifty-four-year-old Denise also described learning how to squeeze her legs together to give herself pleasure as early as seven or eight and soon after how to touch herself in bed to create the same sensation until she reached orgasm:

> I didn't tell anyone except my little sister. I wonder if she remembers. One time, she saw me and asked me what I was doing, and I said, 'It tickles a lot, then it feels like a sneeze, and then a light flashing on and off down there.' In retrospect that's a pretty good description. Then when I found out what it was, I was like, 'Oh my gosh, I've been doing this for years! I had no idea you could do it with another person or that it had anything to do with sex.

How Not to Lose Your Virginity

Returning to my story, one Saturday night when I was 14, a boy who ran in our circles announced that his parents were out of town. Coincidentally, mine were too, and Charlene arranged to spend the weekend at my house which was our usual M.O. When we arrived at the party, Charlene and I were the only girls, and about a half-dozen boys about our age completed the group. I don't remember the host's name, but he had procured a lot of liquor. I also don't recall much about what happened next except that drinking games resulted in everyone being naked. The rest is a blur, but Charlene and I were passed around between the boys and sexually experimented with until everyone threw up or lost consciousness. One of the boys, whose face I vaguely recall due to his flicker of kindness, took a particular interest in me. Somehow I was removed from the party and returned to my house several blocks away.

The following day, Charlene insisted we return to the scene of the crime to help clean up before the host's parents came home. The mismatch of our emotional response to this event was the beginning of the end for our friendship. Charlene appeared proud and victorious, stuffing any shame or pain beyond perception. She insisted she'd fallen in love with one of these boys and wanted to hang out with him the following afternoon. I, on the other hand, was in complete shock. I had no real understanding of what had happened but knew I had crossed a line that I could never come back from. I felt sick, and my head was spinning, a sensation that I now know as being deeply ashamed. My intuition—the wisdom and moral compass that I was born with—knew that something was seriously wrong.

Meanwhile, these boys seemed to like me, and Charlene was pleased with our accomplishments. Having lost the tiny amount of value I had previously placed in myself, I didn't have anything else to lose. So we went back that Sunday. Charlene ended up drunk and in bed with her "boyfriend," and I found myself in the same room with them and the one boy who had claimed me for himself. Luckily, our afternoon orgy was cut short by rumors that the parents were in the driveway, and we all made a hasty exit through the bedroom window.

Somehow, the small-town communication network, fueled by bragging teenage boys, spread the details of this weekend far enough to reach our parents. I desperately wanted someone to do something. Punish me. Send me to counseling. Do something—anything—to keep me from sinking further into this bottomless well of shame and self-destruction. But nothing happened. If they had wanted to do the one thing that would make me feel the worst, doing nothing was it. I wasn't even worth fighting for—not even worth punishing. In reality, my parents were completely ill-equipped to have the conversation we needed to have. My mother went to her room and cut off the small amount of communication she'd previously had with me. My father worked longer hours and drank more. I was completely and utterly alone. Charlene's parents, on the other hand, went ballistic. She was grounded for weeks, and her father threatened to send her to boarding school. I was insanely jealous.

Distorted and Unchallenged

It's hard to re-enter the brain of myself as a teenager without applying the lens and wisdom of the adult, but I think my coping mechanism for making sense of where I was at age 14 was to be pragmatic. I may have been damaged goods, but I was going to make the most of my changed status. Since I couldn't move backwards, I would embrace my new set of circumstances and be better at it than anyone else. I went all-in being the "bad girl," with the exception of keeping perfect grades at school. Although I steered away from the trauma of sex for at least another year, Charlene and I continued to experiment with alcohol, marijuana, partying, and manipulating boys. We never spoke of that weekend again. Without adult wisdom or guidance, I had absolutely no way to process what had happened. It became forever ingrained in my psyche from the perspective of a 14-year-old girl.

What I thought about sex became deeply distorted and unchallenged. Sex was naughty; that was for sure. It got you in trouble but also elevated your status in certain circles. It earned you attention and made boys like you. It was something special that I had done and most people hadn't. I had some secret knowledge that others wanted. The value of sex became entirely a commodity, completely removed from its essence in love and connection. It was a way to get what you wanted, nothing more.

Sex wasn't something girls wanted, rather it was something boys wanted and girls could provide if the situation suited them. It gave girls power over boys. It was mine. I owned it, and I could trade it for love or attention or withhold it as I pleased. For the next 33 years, that is how it remained. I didn't have a real boyfriend until I was 17, and he was my fourth sexual partner. By this age, I had owned my sexuality and proudly displayed it as an "expert," building elaborate walls to protect myself from hurt while proceeding to break hearts right and left. I had learned how to use starvation and physical activity to lose weight. I could manipulate the genetic realties of having curly red hair and an unremarkable face to be pretty. I would date one guy then date his best friend. I was merciless, and I was in charge. The little girl who hadn't been loved and was raped, abused, and neglected devised a subconscious plan to erase all that pain. No one could hurt me. I graduated from high school at the top of my class. I sought to control everything and everyone in my path. Sex was power.

In my 20s, I continued to view sex as a way to attract men and have power over them. I decided when we had sex and how often and used my expertise to keep them around. I often dated men much older than me, including a physically abusive 37-year-old when I was 18 and one of my much older surgical professors when I was 25. The professor was wealthy and took me on romantic getaways to faraway places and foolishly got me highly visible front-row tickets to sports games and introduced me to the players. All I had to do was look sexy and perform in bed. He was later fired as a result of the affair.

Sex was exciting and on the edge of dangerous. Once I was arrested for having sex in public. It was actually in the middle of a nature reserve. The only person who saw us was the police officer, but he was apparently offended. There were plenty of other times I didn't get arrested.

Megan had a similar story and relates:

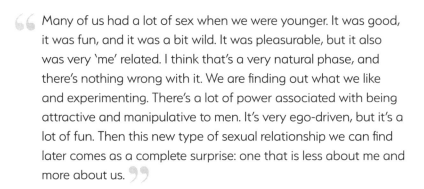

> Many of us had a lot of sex when we were younger. It was good, it was fun, and it was a bit wild. It was pleasurable, but it also was very 'me' related. I think that's a very natural phase, and there's nothing wrong with it. We are finding out what we like and experimenting. There's a lot of power associated with being attractive and manipulative to men. It's very ego-driven, but it's a lot of fun. Then this new type of sexual relationship we can find later comes as a complete surprise: one that is less about me and more about us.

I wasn't completely detached from my feelings and fell in love more than once, but I met my match with Javier, my senior-year medical school boyfriend. He was a drop-dead gorgeous, magnetically charismatic Peruvian-American several years behind me in school. Javier sang, played the Spanish guitar, lifted weights for several hours a day, and had a certain way of getting out of a swimming pool and slicking back his hair that almost made me faint. He was in control of our relationship for sure, and I followed him along like a hypnotized puppy. Javier lost interest in me after about a year, moved on to a long list of other girlfriends, and finally married in his mid-40s (not that I followed him on Facebook or anything).

After that painful breakup, I was ready to be back in the driver's seat, and the next man I met became my first husband. Conservative, Catholic, and looking to settle down, he was pretty certain to never leave me. On the good side, he was a very intelligent, hard-working attorney from a "Beaver Cleaver" family. This fulfilled my dreams of having a cookie cutter, white-picket-fence home life to replace the disastrous one I'd run away from. My subconscious mind had picked a husband, and he was good breeding material. There was nothing romantic or passionate about it. Still, we initially had a lot of sex. In fact, we had very messy drunken sex on the night of our first date. Not thinking the relationship would last long, this seemed like a good way to move on from Javier and prove to myself that I was over him, particularly since Javier's sister was my roommate and would give a full report to her brother. Note to self: rebound relationships are all about control and manipulation.

Sex, Control, and Manipulation

The subject of women like me using sex as control and manipulation, far removed from its potential as a portal into love and connection, came up over and over again in my interviews. Caitlin describes:

> Sex with my first husband was under my complete control. We did it whenever I wanted to and only when I wanted to. The purpose of the game was for me to have as many orgasms as possible, sometimes up to eight at a time, and we even began referring to orgasms as points. I don't recall caring much at all about what he got out of the whole experience. It was all about me. The other

purpose, of course, was to cast a spell on him that would make him marry me. Being sexy was a big part of that agenda. And after we got married, it was all about getting pregnant. Sex was a game that I was always out to win. It was currency. This is what I had been taught.

When I had long since landed my mate, I had my tubes tied after I'd checked the box of having kids. At that point, sex became completely purposeless. While I still found pleasure with masturbation—on my schedule, when I wanted to, and mostly for stress relief rather than pleasure—having my husband physically close to me became at best an annoyance and at worst completely repulsive. Not only did I not enjoy sex, I hated it and dreaded the inevitability that it would have to be done on occasion to keep us together. I reduced it to the absolute minimum and participated as little as possible to get it over with as fast as possible.

My resentment started to grow and seethe when he would still approach me to have sex despite my obvious lack of interest. All of these feelings were projected onto him until I hated the way he walked, breathed, held the newspaper, and chewed his cereal. We were as disconnected as two people could ever be. I had absolutely no concept of what I was missing. Looking back, I was operating as about half of a person.

Without a doubt, what we learn as a child, both from our primary caregivers and from our early sexual experiences, profoundly shapes the way we relate to sex in the future. While we can't turn back the clock, examining our old conditioning and how it is showing up in our current relationships is vital. It's the first step to awakening into the brave new world of a truly loving, intimate sexual connection that we will soon learn about. Once we really study and get to know ourselves, we can finally understand why our minds operate the way they do, often causing us to speak and act in ways that cause harm to ourselves and others. Only then can we start to live a life of freedom and awakening, no longer being dragged subconsciously around by our less- evolved brain.

FIVE

Who Are We, Anyway?

There's a reason why this book centers on finding and knowing yourself. Midlife is a miraculous time when you have hopefully gathered enough wisdom to tackle this incredibly important project. I have personally experienced finding myself like picking up pieces of a jigsaw puzzle over time, deciding which ones fit and throwing others back. It doesn't happen overnight.

The sexual part of our nature is just one piece of the puzzle, and yet it's one that's often overlooked. But before diving too much into the ultimate goal (in the context of this book) of finding your sexual being, let's talk about the process of finding yourself at all. What does that even look like? More importantly, what does it have to do with sexuality?

Shaped by Childhood Experiences

My life began in New Zealand in a suburb surrounded by farmland. Perhaps you grew up in a bustling, metropolitan city or in a smaller town with an unspoken sense of community. No matter where or how you were raised, your early experiences profoundly shape what you believe and the lens through which you see the world. Your early experiences with connection—or disconnection—through your family, school, church, friendships, and culture frame the world for you. The world becomes either safe or dangerous, accepting or disapproving, loving or neglectful. The process of hardwired "conditioning" starts.

Conditioning is the process of learning how to think and behave based on the conditions to which you are exposed. Since each of us experiences different conditions, we each learn a different "reality" that's pieced together in our brains into something that we believe to be true based on our own unique experiences. This includes what we are taught by example and through experience, as well as everything coming through our senses from our environment. It's like we are all looking at the same reality through a different lens. To each of us, things appear unique.

Back to you. While much of your conditioning is useful—you learn not to put your hand in a fire because it burns—much of it is harmful and can separate us from our longed-for sources of love and connection. In the extreme, if you were taught to believe that others are inferior or dangerous, conditioning can create hate and war. In more subtle cases, it can create the belief that you are not enough or are even innately unlovable. Whatever our conditioning, much of it teaches us the many ways that we are right and others are wrong. It can divide us. In as much as it divides us, it's simply not true. Connection, not division, is at the center of everything I know about what's true and what matters if we want to grow. Division can keep us very, very small.

Examining and unwinding your conditioning starts the process of self-awareness and self-discovery that leads to freedom. Freedom from limiting beliefs that are not true. Freedom from thoughts that keep you disconnected and separated from the love you need. Freedom to be open to reality as it is without the murky lens of unconscious biases through which you view the world. Freedom to be the person you were put here to be: your best, true, and authentic capital "S" Self.

Big Me, Little Me

I often talk about "Big Me" and "Little Me" when teaching or coaching around this concept. I identify Big Me as your best potential Self. She represents the most evolved version of you, with qualities like compassion, creativity, accountability, curiosity, openness, generosity, bravery, kindness, integrity—and add any value that resonates with your heart. Perhaps Big Me is easier to imagine as your ideal "future Self" who operates according to your core values and is someone you are always proud of. Little Me represents your less evolved state, with qualities of fear, self-preservation, victimhood, blame, closed mindedness, and judgmental thinking. In fact, a very basic version of this concept boils down to the spectrum of human possibility from "angel" to "animal" or even more simply, from "love" to "fear."

If you are operating from love, Big Me is driving. Little Me's wheelhouse is fear. Big Me is aware of her own conditioning and is able to pause and bypass unhealthy reactivity, and then respond from a place of wisdom with an understanding that she is the creator of her own path. Little Me is lost in a trance of old conditioning and reacts unwisely without a feeling of choice or accountability, since everything is always someone else's fault. Sound familiar?

Grab Your Shovel and Dig Deep

I mentioned core values above and want to pass on one really effective method at digging into what those are. This is one of the fundamental building blocks in figuring out who you really are and how to show up as your best Self. Why does this matter? Because you can't be present in your own skin, let alone in a genuinely connected relationship, until you figure out who is here. Confession: I really hate books with exercises in them, and I never ever do them. With that said, please try this exercise, which takes just a few minutes, a pen, and a piece of paper.

Here's the CliffsNotes version. Consider the three or four people, living or dead, that you admire the most. Among those three or four may be a prophet, relative, friend, or historical character. Write down their names. Under each name, list the qualities you respect the most about that person. After completing the list, look for similarities in the lists and identify any descriptors that appear several times. It's likely that the most common descriptors represent your core values.

> You can't be present in your own skin, let alone in a genuinely connected relationship, until you figure out who is here.

When I did this simple exercise the first time, I hadn't heard the punch line and was completely blown away when asked to consider that my list approximated my own core values. If the teacher had just asked me to write down my core values, I think I would have been completely stuck. It's usually a lot easier to come to self-awareness by seeing our own values reflected through others.

That fact illustrates how desperately disconnected most of us are from awareness of our own true nature. We draw a blank when we even think about it. At least I did, until fairly recently. But I truly believe we are all doing the best we can with what we were given and the causes and conditions that we were born into. We all suck at self-awareness—until we don't. And no one gets there by accident. If you're reading this book, you are doing the work, so high five yourself for that.

Back to the exercise. My personal list includes courage, kindness, generosity, connection, equanimity (unflappability or balance), self-awareness, and tenacity. When asked to examine which areas in my life reflected these values and which didn't, I was humbled. For the first time, I understood that living authentically meant I would need to examine my old conditioning and make some changes. For example, courage showed up as a core value, yet I was too scared to speak up about my miserable marriage or to have difficult conversations at work. Instead I suffered for years by not telling my then-husband what I really needed. I also talked about people behind their backs instead of confronting them with hard issues at the office. Equanimity and kindness were core values, but I lost my temper regularly and bit people's heads off. Sure, I was kind and generous and courageous most of the time, but authenticity isn't a part-time job.

Interestingly, I realized that whenever I acted out of alignment with my core values, I felt awful. Similar to what Brené Brown famously described as a "vulnerability hangover"—that awful doubt after you have revealed yourself publicly—I would have an "inauthenticity hangover." This would typically happen after I'd spoken up in a high-level business meeting or contract negotiation. I would run over everyone in the room with some version of "my way or the highway," including subtle, socially acceptable threats and bullying to get my way. The outcome was inevitably successful (if success is measured in traditional terms), and my business partners would congratulate me. So why would I leave the room feeling nauseated?

While possibly modeling courage and tenacity, it was not modeled in a way that valued kindness, connection, and equanimity. It destroyed relationships. My gut told me over and over again that something was wrong. It took many, many years for me to listen. This is just one way that listening to your body will impart you with enormous wisdom. Fast forward to the present. If I'm considering whether a decision is in line with my core values, I can pay attention to how my body feels. It's pretty much always right.

I love my teacher Vinny's saying:

 If you want to feel good about yourself, do things that you feel good about. "

When I act in accordance with my core values, I feel good. When I don't, I feel lousy. It's that simple.

Keep Digging

Here's another exercise to help you figure out the "who am I?" question. It involves writing a list of things that are associated with you feeling happy, a description of times you recall feeling deeply content and a description of times you felt deep discontent. This exercise takes quite a bit of time and truly deep reflection. What common elements were present when you felt happy? Or unhappy? For me, as for many, my deepest experiences of contentment were almost always associated with connection with another, of being accepted, loved, and being of value. The overarching feeling of happiness for me is rooted in not wanting anything to be different and being completely present in the moment. It's really the breaks from wanting, as small as they may be, that are associated with peace and contentment for me. Conversely, when I am unhappy, there is something I want to be different, and I am stuck in fighting reality and ruminating on a better past or future.

Tara Brach is one of my favorite authors, speakers, and teachers. She led an exercise with our group at a retreat a few years ago, and it really resonated with me. We were asked to work with a partner and repeatedly ask each other, "What do you love?" At first, the rather low-hanging fruit popped up for me: my family, my dogs, a nice spring day—but after many repetitions, my answers got much deeper. Things showed up like the smell of rain on hot asphalt, the colors of the sky on the beach at sunset, having my head massaged at the hair salon, talking to a homeless person at a traffic light, making an improved protocol or a cool spreadsheet at work, listening to silence in the middle of nowhere, and writing a poem. I suddenly realized I loved so many things. When I reflected on this, patterns began to emerge about the things in life that really resonate with me on a spiritual level, the level of my deepest true Self. This is who I am.

Love, connection, nature, creativity, and service were at the top of the list. I love being with real people in a really genuine way. I love to love. I don't like big cities. I love oceans, lakes, forests, beaches, and animals in their natural habitats. Part of me is drawn to make a mark on the world by creating something new, something that wasn't here before me, by finding and living in my unique genius. I feel called to challenge the status quo and to help move the needle toward a higher evolution. I know I was put here to serve and being of value to others makes me feel natural and at home.

I discovered that I had spent most of my life trying to look like someone I wasn't. My authentic Self loves wearing comfy athletic clothes and minimal makeup. All of the times I recalled being happy had nothing to do with the dress I was wearing. I realized that I love peace. I hate conflict and loud noise unless it's live music. But I also realized that I was pretty committed to conflict in many areas of my life. If you think this sounds like an unfortunate and painful contradiction, you are absolutely right!

I deeply respect the idea from relationship experts Gay and Kathlyn Hendricks' book *Conscious Loving*, that we can find out what we are committed to by examining our results. If we are surrounded by conflict, then we are committed at some level to keeping that conflict going. This was a tough pill to swallow because I liked to think that "I didn't start it," but as a participant, I was clearly committing to keeping it going. What we are truly committed to will show up in our lives by examining our results.

> **What we are truly committed to will show up in our lives by examining our results.**

I seriously hated that sentence for a long time and fought tooth and nail against it. If in fact it was true, then I must actually be responsible for the outcomes in my life. That would be a game changer because I wouldn't be able to blame others for my suffering anymore. I would have to learn a whole new way of being. If you are anything like me, you will deny it with a passion until you can't deny it anymore. What we are truly committed to will show up in our lives by examining our results is just capital "T"

True, and it hurts like hell to accept. I was going to have to examine my old conditioning and change some things to live in alignment with this emerging authentic true Self.

Creating Your Own Destiny

Have you ever had the experience of figuring something out for the first time and then all of a sudden seeing it expressed all over the place? When I accept that something is just True, I have found that it shows up in front of me. Right after I read and finally accepted the Hendricks' wisdom, these same ideas were presented to me by Jim Dethmer and Diana Chapman in their life-changing book *The 15 Commitments of Conscious Leadership*, which explores this same truth from a business and leadership perspective.

The first of the 15 Commitments is to *take full responsibility for every outcome in your life*. Hmmm. I hadn't gone looking for this book, but my practice administrator happened to pick it up by chance simply because she was attracted to the title. As a side note, it now holds the guiding principles for my business culture and coaching practice, and I work with Jim and Diana in person. Less than a month later, I happened to read what is now one of my all-time favorite books, *The Art of Racing in the Rain*, in which the central character, who happens to be a dog, says:

That which we manifest is before us; we are the creators of our own destiny. Be it through intention or ignorance, our successes and our failures have been brought on by none other than ourselves.

— Garth Stein

While taking full responsibility, it's inevitable that you have to look at and let go of many of your old stories. Here's an example of why. One of my stories is that much of my own unhealthy conditioning came from having emotionally disconnected parents who withheld love from me as a form of punishment. My mother, in particular, was emotionally immature, fragile, and ill-equipped to handle the demands of five children. I was regularly left alone when she couldn't cope anymore. Even worse, I became the family scapegoat for everything that went wrong. My mother came to despise me and loved my sisters more. She would separate me from the others by withdrawing her affection from only me. I would be left alone, and she would take the "good children" with her. I reacted by filling the role of being the "bad child," or at least that's the story my childish mind created. I created a single, narrow, and unchallenged story of myself as a child and of my mother, which I carried with me well into adulthood.

Who knows what really happened, since few of our stories are true. But as a result, I created a reality in which something is inherently wrong with me, that people who love me will leave me, and that abandonment is right around the corner, so armoring up to prepare for that probability would be wise. I created a tough exterior to pretend my mother's actions didn't hurt, and I transferred that same belief system to all of my close relationships. I left home and left New Zealand as soon as I could. At the same time, I was being physically abused by a much older man who said he loved me and would simultaneously push, grab, and physically restrain me. By age 18, my story was so ingrained that I was sure it was better to take control and leave a situation rather than stick around and continue to be hurt.

> I never let myself get vulnerable enough to be seriously hurt. I intentionally kept distance and shared very few secrets. I never let him really get to know me, and I never got to know myself.

In my first marriage, this played out as a general lack of connection and a business-like relationship in which I was rarely truly present. I never let myself get vulnerable enough to be seriously hurt. I intentionally kept distance and shared very few secrets. I never let him really get to know me, and I never got to know myself.

Early in my next marriage, this unhealthy conditioning caused us plenty of problems. When we were dating and deeply in love, I would regularly leave in the middle of the night, fueled by an unconscious fear of vulnerability and desire to not be hurt. Later, I would be certain that he was going to leave me and would create elaborate stories in my mind to support my position. Since he was going to leave me, I was going to be ready and was not going to be surprised.

Thankfully, through some deep self-reflection, as well as several insight meditation retreats, a good dose of coaching, counseling, and finally committing to deeply listening to each other, we were able to start rewiring this old conditioning. The key was understanding its source, giving it compassion, and finally letting it go. Perhaps the phrase "just let it be" is more accurate since even when I just "let things go," they still seem to be there. I have lots of old stories and habits that I thought I had "let go," but they apparently didn't get the message and keep showing up. I just don't engage with them anymore. I am the witness, not the actor, in the story, or at least that's the aspiration.

Obviously, a more likely ending to this particular story would be that he would have grown tired of this literally childish behavior and left. This would have validated my delusional belief that everyone who loves you is untrustworthy and leaves, reinforcing the old conditioning even further and ultimately creating a self-fulfilling prophecy. There was every danger of exactly that.

Since we are all living in stories that we create ourselves, we often create the things we fear the most. Since we write the script, the script includes our thoughts and fears. Let's unpack how that works. If you fear abandonment, you often act in fearful or childish ways that push others away, like I did in my story above. If you fear that you're not good enough or something is wrong with you, chances are you'll shy away from opportunities to shine, which allows others to collect praise, promotions, and social status while you don't. Maybe you work tirelessly to be perfect and "better than" to desperately try to prove that nothing is wrong with you. That was my primary M.O., and frankly, it's exhausting and never ever works. Perfectionism is a setup to keep the myth that there's something wrong with you going because you will never be perfect. The inner critic drives the perfectionist who then feeds the inner critic. They are stuck together in a perpetual whirling dance of synergistic misery.

Megan shared a great story of how the self-fulfilling prophecy played out in her marriage to her second husband Rob. Meeting in their mid-40s after respective long first marriages and bitter divorces caused by infidelity, Megan and Rob had learned not to trust and assumed that betrayal was right around the corner. She relates:

 After my divorce, I had a couple of relationships before I met Rob, and while neither one of them worked long-term, we remained friends. Rob and I were deeply in love and felt like soul mates as soon as we met. We had amazing conversations, incredible sex, and loved everything about each other with one exception. Rob hated that I still talked to my male friends even though they, too, had both moved on, and I showered Rob with love, affection, and devotion.

As time passed, I started talking to my male friends secretly because I didn't want to upset Rob but wasn't willing to let go of these important connections. I don't have so many friends that I want to give up people who care about me. One day, Rob caught me mid-conversation, grabbed the phone, looked through my texts and emails, and accused me of being unfaithful. The accusation and the jealousy were so painful that we started to disconnect. We stopped making love. He started going away more for work and often slept in the guest room to have "space." When we were in the same bed, Rob would turn his back and go to sleep.

I was so lonely. I started talking to other friends more and more and began connecting with other people. He looked on my phone and computer regularly and questioned me about my contacts. I felt so betrayed by the privacy invasion that I shut down and told him if he ever did that again, I wanted him to leave. One lonely night after a couple of glasses of wine, I looked on an online dating site just to try to feel connected with someone—anyone—who wanted me. Soon after, I met a guy online and we started talking romantically, eventually met and had a brief affair. Rob found out about that, too, in one of his phone searches and said it was over between us.

I guess deep down I always expected that he would leave me since I thought all men are just not trustworthy and can't commit. My first husband cheated on me, and my father left when I was a teenager. Maybe that has something to do with it. Rob's first wife was an alcoholic and was constantly lying about her drinking and overspending, and he had learned that women were basically deceptive.

After a brief separation, we realized, luckily, that we really wanted to break this cycle and work things out. We saw that we both had acted from old patterns and were able to get counseling, read some really good books, and talk about our triggers openly so we were not harboring resentment. Slowly, we learned to trust again and realized that the basic source of mistrust was from our past, not the present, and that we were both reenacting old dramas.

Megan and Rob realized they'd created what they feared most through their own actions. It's surprisingly easy to make something happen simply by believing it will happen, as their story shows. The good news is that this also works in reverse. In other words, we can create a good outcome with our beliefs as well. As the iconic Mary Kay (cosmetics) says, "Expect great things, and great things will happen."

I think most of life is a self-fulfilling prophecy. In other words, we create our own reality. If you shut down to the possibility that amazing and

> **We create our own reality by simply deciding what we pay attention to.**

miraculous things will happen, then you won't see them or will discard them when they do happen. Sadly, you'll feel gratified in proving that the world is a dangerous and untrustworthy place that basically sucks. On the flip side, if you open up to the possibility that amazing and miraculous things will happen, then your senses will notice when they appear, and you will be proven right that the world is your ally. We create our own reality consciously or unconsciously by simply deciding what we pay attention to. The trick is to move what we pay attention to into consciousness and consciously choose what we pay attention to *very* carefully.

"The most important question you can ask is if the universe is a friendly place. For if we decide that the universe is an unfriendly place, then we will use our technology, our scientific discoveries and our natural resources to achieve safety and power by creating bigger walls to keep out the unfriendliness and bigger weapons to destroy all that which is unfriendly. I believe that we are getting to a place where technology is powerful enough that we may either completely isolate or destroy ourselves as well in this process. If we decide that the universe is neither friendly nor unfriendly and that God is essentially 'playing dice with the universe,' then we are simply victims to the random toss of the dice and our lives have no real purpose or meaning. But if we decide that t he universe is a friendly place, then we will use our technology, our scientific discoveries, and our natural resources to create tools and models for understanding that universe. Because power and safety will come through understanding its workings and its motives."
—Albert Einstein

Someone Has to Go First

While few people would dare to argue with Einstein, a skeptic might suggest that we're simply making up a story to believe in, that the world must be either friendly or unfriendly, and one can't just decide what's true. The point is that in this way we can actually decide what's true. By believing that the world is friendly and approaching people as if this is true, then we will create a friendly world. The other option is to create the end of the world, which sadly seems to be where we are heading currently.

> **If you are waiting for your partner to do something kind and connecting before you respond with kindness and connection, it can be a long and resentful standoff.**

This works exactly the same way in relationships. You generally get back what you put in. If you approach people with openness, trust, and love, you will receive openness, trust, and love back (not always, but usually). If you approach people with aggression, resentment, and lack of trust, you will receive the same. Someone has to go first. If you are waiting for your partner to do something kind and connecting before you respond with kindness and connection, it can be a long and resentful standoff.

Speaking of resentment, through my own experience as well as my interviews and the MRS study, the No. 1 libido killer for women (and probably men) is resentment or unspoken anger. Sophie put it this way:

> I spent my entire first marriage being resentful. I was angry about so many things but had no good way to share my anger and kept it all stuffed inside. Sometimes my anger created so much pressure that it would burst out in scary and confusing ways through tiny cracks in my armor like a soda can opened after it has been shaken. Then I would return to my calm bottled-up state. With no tools to understand a healthy way to release anger, I grew a garden of resentment that was fertilized and watered every day by patterns in my marriage that part of me knew were not in line with my authentic true nature and values, but I could not yet speak about it. Something in me knew that if I started the conversation, our marriage would end, and I wasn't ready for that yet. So I kept my resentment, and my libido was non-existent.

I've heard versions of this story repeated so many times that I've lost count, and it certainly was the case for me in my first marriage. Resentment absolutely kills libido. The kind of sex that takes place in a pool of resentment is certainly not making love. It's sex based in anger, duty, aggression (including my favorite: passive aggression), self-harm, or harm to the other. You can take the word "love" right out of making love and replace it with "fear."

Forgiveness as an Antidote

If I had been a little wiser back then, I would have known that the antidote for resentment is forgiveness. Forgiveness doesn't mean that you believe the other person didn't hurt you or that what someone did was okay. It also doesn't mean that you have to forget. It simply yet powerfully means you are letting it be and no longer recycling those negative emotions. In the words of Reverend Don Felt, "Forgiveness is giving up all hope for a better past."

> Clearing up resentment is absolutely essential if you are going to delve into the world of genuine whole-hearted connections shared by the sexually woke.

Forgiveness will probably require allowing the resentment to first come out as "clean anger"—a healthy way of expressing that you have been hurt without the desire to hurt the other person back and creating new ways to deal with whatever situation made you angry. Without clearing the anger first, forgiveness can be a form of "spiritual bypass" or saying everything is fine when it really isn't, and the anger will come back in a stronger form since it hasn't been processed.

As women, we are taught from a young age not to express anger and that we need to be sweet, nice, and pretty. We are experts at holding resentment. When I think about forgiveness, I think about the prefix "fore" (first) and "giving"—or giving first. Forgiveness truly is an act of generosity and bravery, and someone has to go first. Clearing up resentment is absolutely essential if you are going to delve into the world of genuine whole-hearted connections shared by the sexually woke.

"Anger is a real and valid emotion, billions of years old, intelligently rising in the body to protect us from a real or imaginary threat. Wanting to set boundaries. Ready to say NO. Willing to stand up for our values. Yearning to be heard. Anger is not the problem. Anger is not inherently violent. It is in our REACTION to our anger—that is where the violence begins. When we repress and reject our anger-power, refuse to feel it or even acknowledge it, hide it in order to be 'nice' and please, impress and protect others... when we attack and hurt others in order to find relief from our anger... that is where the 'darkness' lies... in our running... in our disembodiment, not in the anger itself. For there is no true love without love for our anger, when it comes to visit... Underneath the anger, you may just discover a tender, fragile, frightened heart, a beautiful vulnerability... billions of years in the making."
—Jeff Foster

A Kick and a Punch

For the past two years, I have attended a women's yoga and meditation retreat in Ostuni in Southern Italy over the New Year. I know, tough life, right? Our yoga and meditation teacher Federica Clemente—look her up at federicaclemente.com because she is amazing!—is also a highly experienced and incredibly talented Gestalt therapist. Gestalt therapy, highly simplified, focuses on how you are feeling right now rather than investigating the origin of old wounds. We all had lots of fun practicing emotional release by punching and kicking pillows, screaming, yelling, dancing, and crying in various states of undress and performing healing rituals around an altar and a fire. Perhaps this sounds a bit crazy, and in a different era we all would have been burned at the stake. But I found a few sessions of this role-playing and acting out of emotions more freeing than years of traditional psychology and talking on the couch. Anger doesn't go away if we hide it, rather it seethes and grows. To quote Carl Jung, founder of analytical psychology, "What you resist, persists." I am now a big advocate of screaming and punching pillows in a controlled environment. So far, the neighbors haven't complained.

When I mentioned that resentment creates a state of being that's out of alignment with your "authentic true nature," I could almost feel the groan of readers tired of hearing this wishy-washy language with no explanation. Perhaps I am projecting since I certainly tend to roll my eyes when I hear language used this way. So let me attempt to explain. The word "authenticity" has become fashionable lately, and discussion about the quest to discover one's "authentic Self" is almost mainstream. While this is a great development, I for one had very little understanding of the concept until well into my 40s. I remember my father, who after retiring as a depressed family doctor, alcoholic, and heavy smoker, became a Buddhist scholar and teacher, once attempting to discuss with me the age-old "who am I" question. At the time, I was a frantically busy obstetrician with three young children, and he met a quizzical stare.

I had no idea who I was. I could rattle off a series of hats that I wore—mother, wife, doctor, sister, daughter, friend, athlete, leader—but none of them adequately described who I really was inside. I could read my resume and see what I had accomplished, but that didn't cut it either. I recall telling my father that I guessed I was just the culmination of 40 years of conditioning.

Yep, I was the product of my environment combined with whatever genetic inheritance I was born with. I think he said something like, "Hmm, is that so?" or a similarly Zen-type non-answer. I wish my father was alive today to continue that discussion, but it left me wondering and started a path of spiritual curiosity that has guided my life since.

Peeling Off the Layers

Discussing authenticity, as I understand it, first requires an agreement that in our most basic and true nature, we are all pure and good. Underneath all of our conditioning and defenses, each of us is perfect. I absolutely do not believe that anyone is authentically bad.

The brave work of self-awareness and self-discovery requires slowly recognizing and peeling off the protective layers that have been added to hide your authentic self and shield you from danger. It's brave because revealing yourself makes you vulnerable, opens you to judgment and positions you for the possibility that you or others might not like what they see. Besides, if we let go of the story of ourselves, what will be left? This is a primal fear for many, if not most, humans. But if you continually return to a starting point of trusting that your most basic nature is perfect, then revealing yourself will be a lot less scary.

Trusting in basic goodness may seem like a leap of faith if you've experienced the world as an untrustworthy and dangerous place. No doubt, people sometimes do some really harmful things and make some really bad decisions, and all of us have been deeply wounded by other humans. But evidence abounds that humans are good at their core and that when freed from harmful conditioning, we operate from principles of love and compassion. No one is born "bad" or inherently rotten. I challenge you to find a "bad" baby. And no one is beyond hope that they might rediscover their authentic Self in this lifetime.

My son pointed out that in mathematics this is what would be called an axiom, which is an assumption or proposition on which an abstract structure is based. We must believe the axiom to be true for the rest of the system to make sense. Most of mathematics and science is based on axioms. The axiom that humans are basically good at their core is not irrefutable. But if you keep your eyes open, you will witness hundreds of tiny and huge miracles every day, as normal humans perform incredibly kind and loving acts to help others.

> The axiom that humans are basically good at their core is not irrefutable. But if you keep your eyes open, you will witness hundreds of tiny and huge miracles every day.

Watching health care workers come together tirelessly during the COVID-19 pandemic and seeing Houstonians come together to help each other after the devastating floods associated with Hurricane Harvey in 2017, comes to mind immediately. Everyone did something to help. Everyone. More recently, an amazing man named Jared helped me when I was alone way out on a country road on my bike with a serious mechanical problem. Jared spent an hour of his time driving me to a bike shop to get it repaired. As we chatted, I found out that he ran an addiction recovery program, and their refrigerator had just broken. So I went home and bought him one. Miracles can be much smaller and easier to miss, like watching a fellow airline passenger let a flustered mother and baby ahead of him in the TSA line. Or finding a basket of snacks, left by my editor on her doorstep for any visitors to share. Miracles are all around us if we pay attention.

Sure, I could tell a different story. I have traveled many times to work as a volunteer surgeon in Sierra Leone where evidence of one of the world's most brutal, modern-day civil wars is visible everywhere, including an incredibly high percentage of amputees. Amputation was a calling card of the rebel army, routinely using this practice to create terror. Possibly even worse, more than 90 percent of young girls in that country still undergo one of the most barbaric forms of female genital mutilation prior to puberty, despite it being officially illegal.

In our own country, many leading officials model and inspire hate and bigotry. TV news provides a daily reminder of how terribly humans can treat each other and the planet. I've personally been physically, sexually, and emotionally abused, and I've done my fair share of harm to others through unwise words and actions. So who is right? Are we basically good or evil?

I think you get to choose. You choose what to pay attention to. You choose what to think and believe. These words speak volumes:

"Your beliefs become your thoughts,
Your thoughts become your words,
Your words become your actions,
Your actions become your habits,
Your habits become your values,
Your values become your destiny."
—Mahatma Gandhi

If you don't believe me, you might find it harder to argue with Einstein and Gandhi. My teenagers, like teenagers should, argue about everything. They might question, "How can you say that goodness is our basic nature? Why couldn't you just say that evil is our basic nature? Aren't you just making up what you want to believe? Why is that any different than just believing in the Church of the Flying Spaghetti Monster?" I think the answers to those questions go back to the understanding that you create your own reality. If you believe that goodness is your basic nature, then goodness becomes your basic nature. To quote American author James Redfield: "Where attention goes, energy flows."

Circle of Compassion

Here's another cool twist. If we trust that the universe is a benevolent place and that goodness is our basic nature, then it follows that goodness is my basic nature and yours too. It's amazing how talented most women are at excluding ourselves from our circle of compassion. We can be kind to everyone in the world but ourselves, assume the best about everyone while simultaneously beating ourselves up and talking to ourselves with a critical voice that we would never use on anyone else. Many women consider themselves uniquely unworthy of love and compassion. While most agree that compassion is the appropriate response to pain, we treat our own pain with disdain.

> **It's amazing how talented most women are at excluding ourselves from our circle of compassion.**

Here's an idea that is pretty humbling: excluding ourselves from compassion is actually a bit of an arrogant perspective because it makes us special and different from everyone else. We are uniquely and especially worse. But if goodness is the basic nature of humans, and I am a human, then I must be basically good too. What a relief it was when I finally understood that fact after 45 years and was able to include myself in my own circle of compassion. At least sometimes. Even me. Whatever you were told or taught about not being worthy of compassion was passed on to you by someone in pain who had been taught by someone else. But it's just not true.

I have a deep understanding that we are all here to re-discover our best Self within, to put her in the driver's seat and to share that gift of love and compassion with others through whatever our unique authentic genius may be. For some of us, this is sharing our expression though art or music, serving others in any capacity, raising a loving family, caring for our parents, talking with a homeless person, or giving directions to a perfect stranger. However it is expressed, the common thread is that our best Self is always connected with others in love and compassion and has a genuine wish for the well-being of yourself and others. For many of us, it takes until midlife for these lessons to be available to be learned or to have time to even consider them. And there's a lot of relearning to do.

> *"Finding yourself is not really how it works. You aren't a ten-dollar bill in last winter's coat pocket. You are also not lost. You are right here. Buried under cultural conditioning, other people's opinions, and inaccurate conclusions you drew as a kid that became your beliefs about who you are. Finding yourself is actually returning to yourself. It's an unlearning, an excavation, a remembering who you were before the world got its hands on you."*
>
> —Emily McDowell

Authentic or Trendy?

One thing I noticed about the concept of authenticity is that it seems to be frequently confused with the opposite, which is following a trend. When I was a teenager, I had my left ear pierced four times, died my red hair black, drank alcohol, smoked pot, and wore lots of black eyeliner while listening to British rock band The Cure most of the day. I argued that I was just "being myself" when in fact I wasn't being myself at all. I was following a trend, albeit a culturally less accepted one, but certainly I wasn't acting from my heart or expressing anything original. Authenticity should not be confused with conforming to a socially less popular subgroup.

A simple test I have for authenticity is asking whether you care what anyone thinks about what you are doing. Are you trying to conform to a certain standard to please others, or are you truly showing up in the way that feels aligned with your own heart's true calling? I can tell you that as a teen I cared more than anything about what people thought, even if my subconscious goal was to push them away.

In midlife, I feel most comfortable in my own skin when I'm not wearing makeup, my hair is in a ponytail, and I'm wearing pajamas or athletic wear. I feel authentic; I feel like myself. I obviously need to dress otherwise for certain situations since I live in a social world and showing up at a professional meeting in my jammies would probably prevent me from connecting to others. However, I have boundaries that I'm not willing to cross. I won't wear high heels if they are hurting my feet, and I won't wear my hair in a style that requires masses of spray or other products to maintain. I can't stand it, and it's not me. Since I want you to meet and connect with the real me, there are lines that I can't cross.

I can't count the number of times I have shown up as someone else. Whoever met me on those days didn't meet anyone real.

Whenever I go to a formal event, I can't wait to wash my face, put on comfy clothes, and put my hair in a ponytail as soon as I get home. Authenticity also shouldn't be confused with saying or doing whatever pops into your head first or blurting out how you're feeling without a filter. That's not authentic; that's just uncontrolled Little Me, which is the opposite of your true best Self. When my learning partner and I were first working together with this concept, he sometimes said exactly what was on his mind at that moment in an unfiltered and insensitive way, followed by the disclaimer "I don't want to have to manipulate my language; I'm just being myself and speaking my truth." My reactive and not-so-enlightened answer was "No, you're being a jackass."

Your authentic Self is kind and compassionate. If you're speaking with hurtful words, consider digging a little deeper. Granted, kindness isn't always "nice" and may not always be received favorably by the loved one—we all know that real love can be tough love sometimes—but that's different than blurting. Yes, love sometimes needs to wield a sword, but it should not use a bludgeon.

In the final analysis, I don't know much for certain, but I do know that you can't show up as your authentic, wisest, and most loving Self unless you know who that is. That's the first step. And if you want to maximize your happiness on this earth, including in relationships, and especially the most vulnerable parts of your life including the bedroom, it's vital to know who that is.

This is where we may need to get a little help from the spiritual masters, and it is the subject of the next chapter.

SIX

Sex, Spirituality, and Finding Yourself

At around seven years old, I clearly recall participating in the Christmas pageant with a minor non-speaking role as a shepherd. With my head draped in sheets tied with rope and my hand gripping a homemade staff, I felt like part of something bigger than myself. In retrospect that was my first experience with the spiritual world. I was more than just Little Me. I was connected with something outside of my own selfish preoccupations, and it was highly attractive.

The most exciting part of the play was a real sheep, which are as common in New Zealand as cockroaches in Texas. While I'm not sure where they got her, the sheep could have been borrowed from just about anyone's land a few miles away where the suburbs turned into seemingly endless rolling hills of green, sheep-studded farmland. Connecting with nature began to be one of the most important life forces that shaped my path. This deep desire to connect and belong and the often-unconscious pull toward a connection with something outside of and bigger than you, is a mark, I believe, of being human.

When you are seven, the desire to be loved by your primary caretaker and to belong to a group that cares about you is literally based in a life or death instinct. As you mature, the desire to be loved and "belong" can still feel vital. I believe it comes from the deep unconscious spiritual knowing that you are not, at your highest potential, a self-centered individual, separate from others. Something in you knows that we are inherently interconnected. Our ultimate purpose lies in connecting with our highest Self and with other living beings.

Linking Spirituality, Authenticity, and Sexuality

What do spirituality, authenticity, and sexuality have to do with each other? In my experience, pretty much everything. First, let's define spirituality. My favorite definition comes from the book *Braving the Wilderness*:

"Spirituality is recognizing and celebrating that we are all inextricably connected to each other by a power greater than all of us, and that our connection to that power and to one another is grounded in love and compassion. Practicing spirituality brings a sense of perspective, meaning, and purpose to our lives."
—Brené Brown

Notice that there's no requirement in this definition to adhere to any certain religious beliefs or even to believe in God. Brown's definition does not exclude anyone. This is foundational since the basic core truth of spiritual life, in my understanding, is interconnectedness, not divisiveness or exclusion. Spirituality and connectedness are really almost synonymous. Connection with something or someone else, by definition, means that something exists outside of yourself. The space in which you connect is the space of shared humanity and freedom from the false idea that you are alone and separate.

Straddling Two Worlds

This is not a book about religion, but what I love the most about religions is what they share, not how they differ, and what we can learn from them, even if you define yourself as agnostic or atheist. Every religion shares a story of the possibility of becoming your best potential Self while still being in human form. While I make no claims to be a theologian or religious scholar, in my Sunday school understanding of Judeo-Christian theology, the Old Testament notes that God created animals and angels and then created man last. Neither animal nor angel, humans seemed doomed to suffer from the consequences of our bad decisions. In the New Testament, Jesus appeared as God in human form, and in Him, mankind's full potential was realized. This has been an incredible inspiration to billions of humans over the past 2,000 years to awaken to the potential within them.

Buddhist discourses include a similar story of a human who evolved through years of deep study and meditation to fully awaken into a godlike state. The historical Buddha was a human, not a god. (He certainly was not a Buddhist, nor did he call himself Buddha, since these terms did not exist until hundreds of years after his death). At the heart of Buddhist philosophy is the optimistic understanding that all humans have the potential to awaken to their most evolved state. In fact, many men and women have done so since the historical Buddha's life over 2,600 years ago, including many people living today.

Similar to the Judeo-Christian description of humans having one foot in each camp, being neither animal nor angel, the Buddha described an ideal middle path between selfish materialism on the one hand and blind dedication to religion on the other. And as I understand it, the Islamic saying "Praise Allah but also tie your camel to a post" recognizes the innate duality that is inherent in the human condition by simultaneously reaching for God and living in the real world with feet on the ground. We straddle two worlds, heaven and earth, but belong fully in neither. Our true potential lies in the ability to integrate them. In interviewee Victoria's words, "Don't be so godly that you are no earthly good!"

> You cannot authentically connect with anyone or anything unless you are connecting as your Self. Whether you are connecting with God, your best friend, or your lover in the bedroom, you have to fully show up first.

So what does any of this have to do with midlife sexuality? Here is where I hope I don't lose you, so take a deep breath. First, to make this idea land, you will need to grasp and deeply know this intersection between spirituality—the connection with something higher than and outside your small self—and authenticity—finding your true nature and acting from that place. The deep understanding of this concept is based on the fact that you cannot authentically connect with anyone or anything unless you are connecting as your Self. Whether you are connecting with God, your best friend, or your lover in the bedroom, you have to fully show up first.

This is what shaped my understanding of the full potential of midlife to offer a portal into a brave and beautiful new world. As you become more authentic, you shed your rough corners and protective layers to reveal the gem underneath that is already there, and you move from the world of animals toward the world of our highest potential.

That is my belief and my statement of hope for myself and everyone else. Whatever your cultural conditioning or religion, I promise you that no one is excluded from this worldview, which I share with many spiritual practitioners and teachers much wiser than myself. This a book about finding yourself, including the most deeply vulnerable parts that have been buried for many years. For many, there's nothing more vulnerable and buried than our sexuality. The journey from fragmentation to wholeness, from isolation to connectedness, to showing up in the world as a complete human being, fully seen by herself and fully present to others, is a journey like no other.

In my view, the connection that I discovered between this brave journey and sexuality is undeniable. In fact, the idea of this book was born because my sex drive blossomed when I began this path of awakening, and I saw the same pattern in many of my patients. It really happens. And it certainly does not require any religion or belief system; it's inherently human.

From Codependence to Freedom

Going back to Shel Silverstein's *The Missing Piece Meets the Big O*—and if you haven't read it, it takes five minutes, and you won't regret it— learning to roll along by yourself (and to polish off the sharp edges that prevent you from rolling) allows you to participate maturely in a genuinely loving relationship with another complete human being. To do so without clinging and codependence is key. Often misunderstood and incorrectly described, codependence is a singular obstacle to psychological and sexual health in an intimate relationship.

Codependence was originally described in the context of addiction, in which the partner of the addicted person becomes sick as well. Sometimes the codependent person behaves in ways that subconsciously fuel the addiction, particularly by taking on a caretaker or helper role that prevents the sick person from taking responsibility for their own recovery. The codependent partner may benefit from or enable the addict's illness by taking on the role of a hero or martyr, or he or she might wallow in self-pity in the role of victim without taking any action to change the situation. In this way, the addict's partner is also dependent on the addictive substance to keep the relationship going—the two members of the dance are each either dependent or codependent on the substance. This could happen when the wife of an abusive alcoholic continues to blame herself for his behavior and cover up his drinking to keep him from getting angry, or when the parent of an addicted teen continues to bail him out of difficult situations rather than risk facing the problem head on.

The term codependent has since been extended to describe unhealthy relationships in which a partner subconsciously undermines the happiness, spiritual growth, or freedom of the other. Put simply, it is the unhealthy clinging and attachment to another despite their unwise or unkind behavior because you need them to fill something that you perceive to be missing in yourself. Unconsciously you need their behavior to continue in order to fill your perceived role as a victim, villain, or hero. A hero needs a victim to save and a villain to conquer. A victim needs a villain to succumb to and a hero to bail them out. A villain needs someone to blame. These three actors in the "drama triangle" all depend on keeping each other in their small, confined roles. They are all codependent, and if any one of them woke up from the trance, the triangle would collapse.

> Often misunderstood and incorrectly described, codependence is a singular obstacle to psychological and sexual health in an intimate relationship.

Sometimes described as "relationship addiction" or "drama addiction," codependence often shows up as a compulsion to keep the other person from being free to make their own decisions, manipulating them to stay when they want to leave, or otherwise creating a system of mutual "stuckness" that creates a prison out of what could be a life of joy, mutual exploration, and growth. It's inevitably associated with relationship drama and lack of positive change or personal growth. And it quite often involves the intentional prevention or destruction of personal growth in oneself and the other person in the misguided effort to keep the relationship together. I say misguided because the intent is good. We all want to be happy. But by mutually depending on each other for what's needed for happiness, we inadvertently enter an agreement to prevent the other person from having the freedom to become their best Self. That is not love. It's dependence, which is based in fear and compulsion, not freedom and choice.

One really sad way I quite often see this expressed in my practice shows up when an obese woman embarks on the brave journey to lose weight and is systematically sabotaged by her partner. Commonly, if she is successful in losing weight and presents herself more confidently and becomes more social, she also becomes more attractive to others. Instead of being happy for her newfound health and happiness, a codependent partner will find this terrifying. Underneath codependence is an intense fear of being abandoned or not needed.

Maryann describes:

> As long as Darryl and I have been together, the main thing we would do as a couple was eat. Our whole lives revolved around food. Shopping for groceries, cooking, and eating massive meals absorbed most of our time together. When I was pregnant, Darryl gained more weight than I did. Both of us became morbidly obese after the kids got older, and while we knew it wasn't healthy, it also brought us closer together because we understood and literally fed each other's addictions. With Darryl, I felt normal and accepted, and while the rest of the 'skinny world' seemed to look down on us, we each said we loved the way we looked and proclaimed to each other that we accepted ourselves as we were and were happy being fat. Deep down we really hated ourselves, but the two of us together made ourselves believe our own BS.
>
> When I was about 45, my doctor told me that my health was really starting to be affected by the weight, and she recommended bariatric surgery. I couldn't believe it had gotten that bad, but she said I would be lucky to live to 55. Darryl fought hard against the surgery, telling me how dangerous it was, but I went ahead with it anyway. I think he felt betrayed... that he had lost his best friend. I think he was scared to lose our only hobby and shared interest. After the surgery and while I had to be on a really limited and special diet, Darryl would constantly try to tempt me with fattening foods and try to get me to eat more than I should. As the weight came off, he started to get more and more angry and jealous. He would accuse me of looking at other men and tell me that my new

clothes made me look slutty. I started going out with a group of weight loss friends from my support group, and he was insanely jealous. Men started to look at me differently, and I realized that I was actually attractive.

Darryl stopped wanting to have sex with me, saying he hated my baggy skin and breasts. He started hiding his own body, realizing that I might not like it so much anymore. I've lost over 80 pounds in the past two years, and I am literally not the same person I used to be. I was hoping Darryl would come on this journey with me, but he doesn't like this new me. I feel like I am growing and moving on, but he is still stuck. And he wants me to be stuck too. But I see a different way to live now, and I deserve to be happy.

Codependent relationships can present in more subtle ways, for example when a husband wants to pursue a hobby or passion that he loves, perhaps expanding into new social circles, and his wife complains or does not allow it. Any desire to restrict the growth or personal freedom of a loved one I would classify as a subtle form of codependence, and we would be wise to keep a keen eye out for it, asking ourselves some honest questions about our intentions and motivations. In the case mentioned here, the wife is making herself depend on the lack of growth or happiness in her husband. Deep down she is terrified that if he grew and changed or sought his own happiness, he would leave her. Again, you can see fear being sneakily disguised as love.

In her book *Codependent No More*, Melodie Beattie describes a codependent person simply as "one who has let another person's behavior affect him or her, and who is obsessed with controlling that person's behavior." Using that definition, it's easy to see how many of us can fall into a subtle form of this relationship trap. Before I read her book, I had never considered myself to have any codependent traits but boy do I. I had been coaching around avoidance of the drama triangle at work for years before I realized that I was playing in multiple, subtle drama triangles at home.

For example, a few years ago, Jill actively encouraged her husband to retire from his corporate job. He was burned out, they were financially stable, and he could pursue his passion as an artist. While this could be a perfectly healthy situation, the subconscious intention is what makes it sticky. Part of her wanted to be the breadwinner to ensure that he wouldn't leave. His job also caused him to travel much of the week, and now she could have him to herself, not to mention he could help out more at home. In setting up this situation, she not only got to enjoy being the hero by paying the bills and making him depend on her, but she also got to be a martyr when he didn't agree to act like a housewife. After all, he was not privy to her subconscious plan (to be honest, neither was she, since it was subconscious), and he had no intentions of being her housewife.

I could tell a hundred other stories of how I did similarly well-meaning things with my own family. Until I was able to recognize a pattern, learn to stop trying to control people, and stop blaming them when they didn't read their lines correctly for what we now call "The Susan Show," I was stuck in recurring and completely unnecessary drama.

Getting back to sex, how does codependence affect our sex lives? As many of us know, the most needy and unhealthy relationships often start out with passion and fire. We have found our long-lost other half, the one who completes us, and it feels euphoric—until we start to feel pain without them, fear they will leave, and try to control them. No longer is sex based in love, compassion, and freedom, but in neediness and compulsion.

Letting Go of the Life Raft

So how do you know if you are in a codependent drama triangle? Check your deepest intentions. I don't know any other way to do that than by sitting quietly and having a very open and honest look at yourself. Do you sometimes feel like a victim (the world is happening to you) or a hero (you swoop in to rescue capable people, often when you don't really want to and they didn't ask)? Do you blame others and cast them as the villain or persecutor in your story? Do you continuously want others to change and feel like they are the problem? Are you more committed to being right than being curious and open? For the record, I do these things all the time!

So finding yourself in a drama triangle, can you allow all of your feelings to be there, letting go of all of your stories of who did what to whom and the way things should be, and recognize the part of you (or the persona) that any unpleasant feelings of injustice come from, and that she is not you? I call that process meditation, but you can call it contemplative prayer, self-inquiry, or just pausing and reflecting. And remember, there's nothing wrong with you. If you are codependent like me, you are a helper, and you mean well, but it's just not working. So give yourself a hug and a breath of acceptance, and decide to make a change. You did the best you could.

In my experience, the cure for codependence is letting go. Or as I said earlier, maybe more accurately "letting be." This is easier said than done after a lifetime of clinging to other humans like life rafts, and it may take as long to undo as it did to create. But it's worth a try for sure, and our happiness ultimately depends on it. Letting go of someone doesn't mean they will leave or that you want them to leave. In fact, it can mean quite the opposite. Letting go of controlling and clinging behaviors that come

> Letting go of controlling and clinging behaviors that come from fear, not love, allows the relationship to be free to blossom and expand.

from fear, not love, allows the relationship to be free to blossom and expand. Love comes from the genuine desire for yourself and the other to be free to become their best Self, possibly together or possibly apart. As Sting so wisely sang about, if you proclaim to love someone, you must set them free. Two free humans who are joyful and growing may then choose to be together in marriage or partnership out of free will, not compulsion.

Carla spent five years figuring out how to make this work in her new marriage. Many times, she thought it wouldn't. More than once, he left, and she didn't think he would come back. Loving someone isn't always easy. Being free and being in a partnership seems like an oxymoron. It's challenging and takes daily—sometimes hourly—check-ins to make sure that your motivation is coming from love, not clinging or codependence.

How do you blend your desire for precious time together with your individual needs to spend time alone? How do you wholeheartedly support the other person in their own journey when it sometimes feels scary and you need support too? This is the balancing act that can make magic or disaster out of a relationship. Trust me, I have had my share of both, but I am finally learning that it is a choice. I understand that I have the power to create balance or destroy it, and currently I choose the former in my relationships. As described by author and relationship psychologist Gay Hendricks, this is moving toward *co-creation*, not codependence.

Here's an example. Last year I went on a writing retreat to attempt to finish this book. The kids were all at camp, and I had two weeks of free time, providing a perfect opportunity for a much needed vacation or a perfect chance for me to go away alone and write. You can feel the setup. It's a great foundation for a massive fight and all kinds of arguments about priorities. What's more important? A vacation or your damn book? And how am I ever going to finish this damn book if I can't ever get a break from work and the kids? Sure, I'd love to go on an expensive vacation, but someone has to work to support the family. Blah blah blah. A few years ago, I would have gone right there, right to the bottom of that rabbit hole, and likely would have spent that two weeks in resentment and blame, doing something I felt wasn't fair, feeling unsupported and unloved, and or feeling guilty and misunderstood.

This is what I did instead, and I can tell you that over time, it starts to become easier and more instinctual. Sitting quietly and connecting with my body by following my breath, I asked myself, "What is the best thing I can do for myself right now? What is my heart calling me to do? Which course of action will help me to feel happy, fulfilled, and create benefit, not harm?" Pretty quickly, the thought of going on a retreat to write and meditate filled my body with a sense of peace and relaxation. It made me smile.

The thought of going on vacation when the book was overdue made me tense, anxious, and overwhelmed. The writing retreat was not just the best thing for me. It wasn't selfish. It was the best thing for my family because relationships will only thrive if each of us is free to follow our own calling. This concept is called "sympathetic joy" in the Buddhist tradition, which is probably one of the most advanced human practices available to us. I admit it continues to be extremely challenging for me.

In Rosie's words:

> The really nice thing is that since the kids have been gone, both of our lives have become freer together as well as apart. There's a whole lecture series he wants to go to. That's fine with me, but I'm not interested. Go learn about World War II submarines. I'd rather not. If I want to go out with my girlfriends, he's cool with that. There's an honoring of the person as a whole person.

My friend was recently divorced, and her ex-husband was a jackass. He controlled everything she did. She couldn't go out to dinner without permission. I could never be in that type of relationship, but I guess when you're in it, you can't imagine what I have. I can make grown-up decisions without having to consult my husband unless it's really going to affect him. I was like, 'I'm going on a cruise with some friends,' and he said, 'Wow, that sounds great! Take some good pictures.' It's not that we don't care what the other does; it's quite the opposite. We love to see the other person exploring and being happy. Then when we get together, we have two happy, whole people.

Genuinely experiencing joy for another person's happiness is not instinctual, even if it is your partner, and particularly when it involves them having happiness without you. When another person experiences success or happiness, how often are you genuinely joyful for their good fortune, or how often do you shrink into jealousy and fear, asking yourself, "Why do they have that, and I don't? That should have been me! What's wrong with me? Why can't I be happy like that?" Even harder to admit, how often do you feel pleased when you see another person fall from the pedestal, lose something that you were envious of, or have some other misfortune?

After my divorce, I'm ashamed to admit that I was secretly happy to hear when other people had relationship problems or separated from a spouse. I definitely didn't want to go to a wedding or hear about someone else's amazing love story. I would think to myself, "There's no way it will work. They'll be divorced in two years." I actually wanted them to fail. When you are suffering, it's often human nature to want others to suffer too.

One of the greatest gifts I've ever given myself was to learn how to observe and choose to step out of this dark world based on fear and scarcity. This is not to say that I don't still have those feelings occasionally, but I can see them as they arise and make a choice to shift toward sympathetic joy. It would be easy to be trapped in a codependent cycle where my partner can only be allowed to be happy with me because if he's happy without me, then he might leave. How insane, when you dissect it, to wish for our loved ones to be unhappy without us. Once again, this is fear cleverly masquerading as love.

Mammals seem to be inherently set up for codependence by the universe's funny joke of giving the woman a hole and the man something to fill it with. But by being gifted as the only self-aware mammals, perhaps part of our destiny is to comprehend and transcend our biological patterning for codependence. Not that we're doing a great job of it. Thousands of songs, poems, and pieces of jewelry play into the addictive and immature delusion that we need another person to complete us. Trust me, approaching relationships from this perspective is likely to have a fiery beginning and an ending that's fiery, feeble, or less than fulfilling. Only two whole humans can coexist in a truly balanced, loving relationship, even if one does have a body part that fits neatly into the other.

> It is only through the long and often painful journey to rediscover your perfectly whole Self, who already exists under a lifetime of misperceptions, fixed views, and habitual conditioning, that you can find the deeply whole and sexual being whose life purpose is to express herself through love and connection.

It is only through the long and often painful journey to rediscover your perfectly whole Self, who already exists under a lifetime of misperceptions, fixed views, and habitual conditioning, that you can find the deeply whole and sexual being whose life purpose, I think, is to express herself through love and connection. There's so much suffering associated with codependence or clinging. For some of us, it might be the only way we have learned to relate to the world and others, and it feels perfectly normal. Even if life feels like perpetual drama and misery, after a while it can become comfortable. But for sure it's not optimal.

Let's face it. Our culture doesn't talk much about wholeness and satisfaction with the way things are. The perception that we constantly need to be fixed or improved keeps our economy going. Being peaceful and content is bad for business!

Cleaning Out the Attic

But what if none of us needs to be "fixed," and we are already whole, even if we can't quite see it? To get there definitely can feel like a struggle, like swimming against the stream. From the day you're born, messages regarding sexuality are constantly drip-fed to you in complex layers of denial, repression, not enough, evil, bad girl, performer, pleaser, danger, power, and manipulation. It's no wonder that our true nature, which I believe comes from love and connection, frequently gets stuffed in a box somewhere deep in the corners of the attic along with all the other things we can't discuss.

Trust me, no one wants to go into the attic. "Demons" of compulsion drive you to behave harmfully and unwisely from old conditioning. Inner critics whisper that you're not good enough. Personas pop their heads out now and then to tell you their cruel and unwise opinions or conversely to give you a glimpse of your true nature on your best days. The hope of fully authentic womanhood can be crushed or intimidated by these demons, or it can be stuck in battle fighting them. You can feel like you're at war with yourself. The person you're trying to let go of constantly derails the person you aspire to be.

Here's an example of how this works for me. A few years ago I gave up delivering babies. It was a tough decision, not only because I loved it and it provided financial stability but also because it had become a deep part of my identity. For a long time I didn't know who I would be if I wasn't an obstetrician. My wise, best Self knew that it was more important to spend time with my family and pursue other passions that were calling me, but my inner critic was certain that I was being lazy, that I would no longer be respected and revered by patients and other doctors, that I would regret it, and that my self-worth depended on me continuing my old career. This is where listening to your heart or gut really comes in to play. When I moved from the endless arguments in my head down into my body, it was impossible for me to ignore what felt right, and I was able to act from my heart and make a change

> You can feel like you're at war with yourself. The person you're trying to let go of constantly derails the person you aspire to be.

with confidence. But it's not easy, especially if this is all happening at a subconscious level. We are simply unaware. Before we can do anything, we need to bring this whole conversation into consciousness.

The work of integrating all parts of yourself and living fully as your authentic Self isn't about defeating your demons, stuffing them back in their attic box, and nailing the lid shut, although that's actually a common strategy. I practiced and mastered it for years and could challenge anyone in the demon-stuffing Olympics. Instead, becoming your Self is about seeing clearly what's there and accepting all of it. It means turning the lights on in the attic, unpacking the box, and having a conversation with everyone and everything there. It's not pretty. In fact, it's messy, and some of them don't talk nicely. But only from that point can you move forward in the light with no secrets, no shame, and a clear understanding of who is in charge. Along those lines, here is another one of my favorite quotes:

"We don't become awakened by imagining figures of light, but by bringing the darkness into consciousness."
—Carl Jung

Who's in charge once the attic box is opened? The fear of letting the inmates run the asylum is profound. Like countless others, it kept me firmly entrenched in the "don't do it" camp for many, many years. I was terrified of losing control, and I did lose control many times, which felt unpleasant, validated my fear, and taught me not to do it again. I think many of us stop there which makes perfect sense. But only by pushing past this initial resistance to discomfort and daring to take the first step toward the process of integration could I ever experience a full life as my true authentic Self—my best aspirational Self—the one I was born as and am destined to return to. That's who is in charge. But let's be very clear: She's not in charge all the time, rather it's an aspiration. I have a keen understanding that she belongs in the driver's seat, even when she has been replaced temporarily by someone less wise.

Who's Behind the Wheel?

I really love the analogy of the driver of a bus or the pilot of a plane controlling our behaviors. In Western culture, being "driven" is used frequently as a compliment to describe someone with a strong work ethic who gets stuff done. For years I was driven, and it made me extremely successful in traditional terms. I rose to the highest levels of the American dream by beating myself like a slave. Then one day I asked myself, "If I am being driven, who is driving? What outside force is telling me what to do? Who is the me in this question? How can I regain my power and drive myself?"

Oxen are driven, herds of sheep are driven, and slaves are driven. Finding our Self means putting her in the driver's seat of our lives and not letting someone less wise do the driving.

"In truth our Self is the ocean. The demons, inner critics, and passing emotions are the waves. And the irony experienced by countless spiritual seekers and prophets from every religion is that once we find our true Self, we live in a world in which we can finally see what has always been there, that our Self is inextricably interconnected with all other beings. Ultimately, we loosen our attachment to Self and become one with everything."
—Taranatha

If this all sounds like tree-hugging nonsense, there actually is a growing body of science from highly respected neuroscientists who are providing hard-to-refute evidence that this is true. To simplify, my own conceptualization of this system is an anatomically top-down approach. Rather than a traditional and typically patriarchal model of spiritual evolution being an upward path toward a heaven in the sky or a mountain top, my view is a downward journey inward from the highest, most recently evolved part of the brain down into the innermost parts of the brain and body, or from the waves down into the depths of the ocean.

Our language seems to universally recognize this progression. We refer to people as "deep" or "shallow" and "airheads" or "grounded." People who are easy going, stable, and self-aware are labeled "down to earth," and those who are stressed out and selfish are "high-strung." There seems to be some communal "knowing" about this concept that many of us have forgotten. We are all too busy trying to get somewhere, and we spend little time being where we are.

Finding yourself involves shifting your attention from your thoughts downward into your body. I have personally experienced that when my mind and body are connected, my center of being sits somewhere right around my heart. I can feel it to the left of center in my chest. From this state of mind-body connection, I can truly be present in the space between myself and others. This is where genuine loving connection takes place with others. It's not a connection of prefrontal cortices; it's a connection of hearts.

Me and We Together

Dr. Dan Siegel brilliantly discusses in his book *Mind* that our mind exists both inside and outside our skull and skin and that connection is a process of energies meeting in the space between us. He defines the mind as a process of energy and information flow that exists both within our skull and skin and in relationship with others. He beautifully defines this blending of self and other in relationship as "Mwe" (neither me nor we, but both together).

In this model, the Ego—synonymous with Little Me or our overthinking mind—is the concept we have of our identity: mother, doctor, author, triathlete, person who owns things that are hers, has a history made up of countless things that happened to her, and is separate and different from any other being. The Ego exists or is felt in the brain, or at least mine is. She thinks incessantly and is always trying to get ahead, rationalizes, and makes up stories, then repeats them over and over again to create a sense of identity. This identity is a collection of Ego-serving stories that have been told so many times that they are accepted as the truth. In all of my stories, the main actor is me. Everything is seen through my narrow point of view, and in every story my role is some version of victim, hero, or villain.

The Ego isn't bad. In fact, you need an Ego to operate, to be able to speak using the words "I" and "me" and to walk around and get things done. It's a part of you that is necessary for survival. But the Ego needs to take her proper place. To quote Robin Sharma, "The mind [Ego] is a wonderful servant but a terrible master."

In contrast, the Self or "Big Me" is generally sensed in the body. This is why body awareness training through yoga, martial arts, meditation, or contemplative prayer, as examples, can be so foundational to the self-awareness journey. And it's also why practitioners of these techniques frequently feel a sense of freedom and connection with others—freedom from the oppressive squeeze of the Ego.

Self or Not-Self?

Maybe all this "becoming one with the universe" talk is making you roll your eyes, but I am really just talking about connection. Connection is inextricably involved in fulfilling relationships and great sex, and we all want those, right?

I didn't make this stuff up; it's been true forever. As my teacher Vinny was once told by his teacher, *"All wisdom is plagiarized. Only your ignorance is original."* While many sources have addressed the importance of connection through losing focus on our small self, these two are particularly poignant:

"To study the self is to know the self; to know the self is to forget the self."
—Dogen Zenji, 13th century Zen master

"If your first concern is to look after yourself, you'll never find yourself. But if you forget about yourself and look to me, you'll find both yourself and me."
—Matthew 10:39

The deep and stable ocean-ness of our being, as opposed to the ever-changing waves, is a space shared by every Self. We might access this space through mindfulness practices, meditation, prayer, service work, or when witnessing everyday miracles like birth, death, or natural beauty. Not surprisingly, this is the space in which falling in love and truly intimate sexual experiences happen and where the landscape is literally made of true belonging and connection.

Dan Siegel calls this space the "plane of possibility." The concept of Not-Self or Me doesn't mean you don't exist as an individual because of course you do. But it points to the observation that nothing about your identity is fixed or solid and that you are constantly changing, even though it doesn't feel that way to the Ego. In moments of connection with people or forces outside of yourself, we universally seem to feel as one. And listen closely: The space in which we connect is not inside your skull. We connect in the space between us, the magical shared space of love and interconnection. So it seems to be a great idea to devote effort to spending more time there. This is not a dress rehearsal. As poet Mary Oliver asks, "Tell me, what is it you plan to do with your one wild and precious life?"

> The space in which we connect is not inside your skull. We connect in the space between us, the magical shared space of love and interconnection.

When I was about 18, I clearly remember reading the Scott Peck classic *The Road Less Traveled* in which he described falling in love as the temporary collapse of Ego boundaries. In this paradigm, the Ego is the selfish, self-referential, and defended small self, obsessed with getting what it can for itself and protecting itself from harm. Letting go of the Ego feels wonderful. Falling in love feels like freedom. No longer are we confined by the Ego's walls, and we seem to melt into the loved one.

I was initially angered that Peck minimized my profoundly unique and special teenage love affair. His paradigm made my experience nothing more than the common, ordinary, and temporary release of my Egoic defenses, allowing me to feel temporarily and completely connected with another. After a while, I understood Peck was right.

Dropping Boundaries in Exchange for Euphoria

Falling in love is entering the ocean-ness of our shared human experience with another person. We have a real and profound experience of being interconnected, and it feels really, really good. Despite being paired with another, we feel completely free. And indeed we are free—free from the Ego's incessant squeeze that keeps us small. Finally, we are free from our small preoccupations and the delusion that we are alone. What a relief! Not infrequently, the loss of Ego boundaries is associated with lots and lots of great sex. Drugs like Ecstasy (MDMA) and Ayahuasca, as well as certain meditation practices, also can create a temporary collapse of Ego boundaries which feels incredibly euphoric. While dropping our Ego boundaries is scary and makes us vulnerable, just like falling in love, it also is very, very attractive. We might have a feeling of being inseparable, of completing the other, or having found our one sure path to happily ever after. We crave it, but there's a major problem: we don't seem to be able to hold onto it.

As we all know and Dr. Peck describes, the Ego sneaks back in disguised as defenses against this highly vulnerable state as the love affair progresses. The peak love experience morphs into a relationship between two defended Egos who at best might genuinely connect once in a while. At worst, they take up arms and actively harm each other. We retreat back into our own camps and put up walls. These walls often run right down the middle of the bed.

Two defended Egos don't make love. They might have sex, but it's not the sex of connection. It's the sex of selfish pleasure, manipulation, duty, or power. Defended Egos usually have sex with the lights off, metaphorically and often literally, and frequently not even with the person in front of them. Defended Egos may require a good dose of alcohol, pornography, checking out altogether by watching TV, or making a to-do list while counting down until it's over. On the animal-angel spectrum, this is way to the left.

The Ego cannot stand vulnerability, which literally means being open to being harmed. This is understandable because the Ego's primal role is to defend us from harm, but without vulnerability, there can be no true connection. How can we truly connect with our armor up? There's no way in. There's no way to connect. The Self remains unseen behind dark walls.

> Without vulnerability, there can be no true connection. How can we truly connect with our armor up? There's no way in.

Maria described her first marriage of 25 years with a man who never showed his true Self and never saw hers. He was conditioned by a strict Catholic upbringing to be disgusted by the naked body, so he never saw her undressed in all those years. Sex was always in the dark, in missionary position, without foreplay, and lasted about 30 seconds. There was no consideration of her pleasure. She never had an orgasm except through masturbation. In 25 years, Maria was never really seen by her husband:

> He was the type of guy that if I wore a nice negligee, I had to change because he said only women from the streets wore stuff like that. Being naked in our own room, as simple as that, was not okay. He always wanted me to be covered.
>
> I felt like I was in prison because I wasn't even allowed to have a credit card in my name. He had control of everything. For the last 10 years of our relationship, I felt like another piece of furniture in the house. I was very angry and frustrated because we couldn't talk about sex. I could not tell him how I felt, and he made me feel like I was the problem.

On the other end of the spectrum of possibilities, the sexuality of our true nature is a pure expression of love, giving, and receiving freely from the undefended heart and experiencing the delight and bliss of union with another. It's a generosity practice, not a "get what I want for myself" practice. In a balanced relationship, the generosity will be returned and will continue to nourish itself. In its highest form, generosity becomes an expression of the ocean—the deep reality that you are not alone. It's a portal into that space of genuine connection, love, and contentment.

Remembering that you are not and have never been alone and that you are inextricably connected by our shared humanity comes with an enormous sense of relief. You don't have to do all this by yourself. Whether with a partner or with yourself, sex in its purest form lets you touch the divine. You can experience the true interconnectedness with another being and through that, a portal to the understanding of interconnectedness with all beings. In that space of connectedness we are free. Free from conditioning and available to be our best Self. Free from the oppressive lie that we are a solitary and self-reliant being. So saying that sex has the potential to be a spiritual experience is undeniable. That is why my work and the thread of everything I know and believe about sex are hinged on that understanding.

Obviously there are other portals into this insight of interconnectedness, but this one doesn't require becoming a nun or going to live in a cave or an Ashram. Quite possibly it's sitting right next to you.

Maria finally got the courage to leave her first marriage after the children left home. When she fell in love with her current husband Max, she said she felt like a virgin. Everything was new:

> I felt awakened and free. Everything looked different and beautiful, like I was seeing things for the first time. I would say, 'Look at this! Look at that!' My life, my soul, my mind were all connected and fully present.
>
> Max taught me about sex because I had never done most things before. Sexuality for Max and me is a part of who we are. It's an energy that flows between us. My understanding now is that through true love, we're able to become our best Selves. He brings out the best in me, and I bring out the best in him.
>
> Before, I was half asleep, like I was in a fog or a daydream. You know in fairy tales how the prince kisses the princess and wakes her up? It's like that, right? She was asleep, and then love woke her up. I think that's where these stories come from. Maybe you can give that love to yourself, or it can be the love of God if you believe that, but without love, you are like a flower without water. I was taught that sex was a sacred gift from God, but I never understood that until Max.
>
> There was no love before. When you really love someone, and they love you, it's like you see yourself mirrored in them. We are separate but also connected, so if he is that amazing, then I know I must be. Love literally wakes you up.

Sixty-year-old, married Episcopal Priest Linda puts it this way:

> On a professional level as a priest, I think that Episcopalians are all about sacramentality—the outward visible signs of internal and spiritual grace. I come to know Christ in you, in the partnership. Marriage is a sacrament in our tradition because of that sense of knowing the holy in myself through you. Your love for me shows me the holy in me, and my love for you shows you the holy in you. There's a transformative potential.
>
> In sacramental theology, you wouldn't just be in love with each other. There's always a sense of the third: what we are producing out of our love for each other. One of the things you might produce is a child, but that's only one of the things. Ideas... creativity... from a theological perspective, sexuality should be generative. It's not just about the two of you. God is in it because there's energy

coming out of it, not just for you, but also for the world. Sex can be an experience of the transcendent that is transcending our bodies and ourselves. We're experiencing it in our bodies, but in the sexual encounter, there's also an opening up beyond oneself and beyond one's body. There's a sense of encountering the transcendent where you are in your body but out of it at the same time. I think orgasm is like that. It's a different type of communion. In a Christian context, you are taking another body into your body. 〞

The Body as a Slave

At this point, I have to admit the irony of reaching this understanding is pretty glaring after a lifetime of studying science, believing the American College of OB/GYN was God and thinking sex was just to make babies, control people, be likable, and fit in. As a scientist, I needed to have an answer to everything. Being right was valued above all else. If a fact couldn't be proven with a randomized controlled trial, it wasn't worth its weight. But this was a brave new world where knowledge came from experience, from the heart, or from a power outside myself (and not from a study or a textbook). It was a whole new way of being. I had to trust my own experience of the truth without validation from outside. This is what Pema Chodron calls "Unconditional Confidence." Maybe others would call it faith. But for sure, it wasn't what I had been conditioned to believe.

As I mentioned, the entire concept of finding oneself went right over my head until I was in my early 40s. I was certain it was a topic reserved for weird yoga hippies who didn't know anything about science. After all, I was a scientist, a surgeon, and a dedicated practitioner of evidence-based medicine. I was also highly experienced at treating the body as something to be beaten into submission and fixed. If it wasn't working, I was trained to cut it, drug it, or otherwise conquer it. There was no accepting anything or discovering any wisdom from the body in this paradigm. The body was a slave and was simply employed by the brain to move it around. The body needed to look good and feel good. It was not supposed to complain, and any pain or suffering was supposed to be either ignored or eradicated quickly by any means possible.

Unfortunately, this is the world of traditional medicine in which all discomfort, change, or other surprising or unpleasant messages from the body are fought against with the passion of an army at war. But being at war with your own body is one of the greatest sources of disconnection from yourself. It cuts you off from one of your greatest—dare I say your very greatest—sources of wisdom.

While Western medicine and culture place enormous value on the analytical mind and very little on the wisdom of the body, this is not a universally accepted scheme of things. Eastern spiritual traditions and all holistic bodies of wisdom recognize that disconnecting the head from the body limits human potential. The body, our "gut feelings," "heart feelings" and intuition—all felt in the body but actually originating in the limbic brain—are often a greater source of wisdom than the thinking mind.

The Full Spectrum of Joy and Intelligence

Finding your authentic true nature inevitably involves sitting still, quieting the mind, listening to what your body is telling you, and treating your body as an ally rather than an annoyance to be controlled. Sexual pleasure may be one of your primary portals into the world of the body's wisdom. Without a mind-body connection, you are surely missing out on enjoying the fullness of sexual experience, as well as the full spectrum of joy and intelligence that the connected mind-body has to offer.

Having a mind-body connection requires having your mind and your body in the same place at the same time. This sounds obvious, but most of us spend very little time being present. Most meditation techniques start with returning attention to the body, often the breath since it's reliable, or another physical cue to remind you to come home. Much of the time, our minds are chasing pleasure or pushing away pain, fantasizing about past and future. Being present is sitting in the middle ground between these extremes, observing without the push and pull. I certainly don't get there all day, but when I do, it's incredibly peaceful!

That doesn't mean that we should give up joy or sadness and be neutral, unfeeling blobs, far from it. When we can be present with our joy and pleasant sensations, we can experience them fully and love every second, knowing that it won't last but not miss what's happening by worrying that it will end. I can't count the number of times my mind has ruined a perfectly wonderful moment. When things are really great, it only takes a second for my mind to start creating a problem. I can be on a dream vacation, and my mind will divide the time in half so I know when we are more than halfway done. After the halfway mark, the dread of the impending last day slowly starts to increase. Typically, the last day of vacation is already consumed with thoughts of leaving. Many of us feel the same way on Sunday evening. In our minds, it's already Monday, and we ruin a perfectly good Sunday.

Here's another way this can go. When things are really great, and I am feeling super present, maybe I am making love or feeling completely connected cuddling and watching a movie, my mind might decide it will be this way forever. I have finally found the answer to everything and will live in perpetual bliss. Then something happens to break the spell, maybe a disagreement or an unwanted interruption from the world—and now I'm resentful and disappointed. It takes A LOT of practice to allow myself to fully experience joy without it morphing into clinging. It's not the joy that's problematic, rather it's clinging to something that by its very nature is impermanent.

The same goes for unpleasant emotions. In and of themselves they are not a problem unless we fuel them by pushing them away or devoting energy to wishing they would be different. My teacher Vinny put it this way:

> I find when I keep things [like painful emotions] under the radar, rather than going away they continue to be there. They cannot die because I have never allowed them to be born. There's part of me that I can't look at because I am pretending it's not there. But if I allow them to exist and come into awareness, they live a natural life and die like all things do.

So when it comes to love and sex, there is a middle ground between the unsustainable peak experience of falling in love and the pain and disconnection of broken hearts and loneliness. I believe this is the promised land of enduring love and sexual well-being. In this middle ground, we can fully experience all of the incredible emotions and pleasurable sensations that are true blessings, and we can do so without either cutting them short or trying to elope with them but still deeply understanding that they are impermanent. Fully immerse yourself in joy and sexual pleasure, and allow yourself to deeply feel life's sadness. The challenge is to see clearly, wake up fully, and understand where you are and what is here. Then start exactly where you are with full acceptance.

As Buddhist monk Ajahn Sumedho popularized, "Right now it's like this." In this space you can agree to disagree with your partner without drama. A disagreement isn't the end of the world. If you are both fully showing up, you won't always see eye to eye since everyone has unique conditioning and experiences. In a healthy relationship, you are two individual, fully formed people, so of course you won't always see things the same way. But without drama, without a victim and a villain, or needing to be right, you can still remain connected and not build that dreaded resentment. If there's one takeaway from this book, it's that resentment kills connection.

Importantly, your own journey toward sexual healing or putting Humpty Dumpty together again does not depend on a partner. More than 1 in 4 women have suffered sexual trauma, and 100 percent of women have experienced other harmful conditioning, so we have a lot of healing to do. But it does not depend on what a partner thinks, says, or does. It's our own work to do alone first. As much as we might want someone else to fix us, they can't. If you are extremely fortunate, you may have a partner who is willing to go on this journey alongside you, but it's not required.

> Only a whole, self-aware person can genuinely connect with another whole, self-aware person without clinging, codependence, and replaying unhealthy past dramas.

Only a whole, self-aware person can genuinely connect with another whole, self-aware person without clinging, codependence, and replaying unhealthy past dramas. There's a reason why we often experience the same problems and dramas in multiple relationships. We take ourselves with us wherever we go. If we haven't done our work yet, we will keep showing up with the same unresolved issues.

If sex is still just a contract to you, or maybe worse, if it's a source of deep pain, trauma, and disconnection, then what I'm saying probably seems kooky or invalidating. It may be deeply out of line with the reality of your experience and may even make you feel worse about yourself or not good enough. I hear you. If you prefer to have sex in the dark with clothes or makeup on, after alcohol or watching porn, or would rather stab yourself in the eye than make eye contact during sex, I get it. I have been there and lived there for all but the past few years. I've also sat with thousands of women who feel the same way.

For most, sex is not a spiritual experience, rather it's a brief, purely physical act that may or may not be enjoyed for a few minutes. Some just tolerate sex while others often dread and avoid it. The question is whether you are willing to take the risk to change that. Through my own journey and through the interviews in the MRS study, I have been part of the most intimate stories of women in midlife who have "crossed to the other shore," not through some magic bullet or potion but by doing the work of deep self-reflection, letting go of old limiting beliefs, stepping out from self-imposed prisons, and learning to live—and make love— with the lights on and with an undefended heart.

Maybe you are wondering why you would ever want to take on such a journey. Maybe it seems too hard, that things are too broken to be fixed, that life would change too much, or that it's just not your lot in life to deserve happiness. For sure, it's not always easy. But I promise you: it is possible.

SEVEN

Pull Yourself Together

N othing has changed my life more positively than realizing I don't have to believe my thoughts. Said differently, I am not my thoughts. This radical idea never occurred to me until my mid-40s. Like most of us, I believed I was my thoughts. In his famous and completely inaccurate 17th century statement, René Descartes said, "I think therefore I am." This summed up the way he, I, and most of us view the thinking mind. As meditation teacher Wes Nisker joked, "Perhaps he should have said 'I breathe, therefore I am.' After all, we can breathe without thinking, but we can't think without breathing." Discovering that my best Self or true nature is actually not my thinking mind changed absolutely everything.

Absent from the Moment

For my entire life, I had listened to my own endless chatter that often seemed to be directing me in several ways at once. I was constantly entwined with myself, with never-ending discussions between the various voices in my head that I just accepted without question. Whatever my thoughts said, I assumed it to be true, and the thoughts never stopped, not even when I was asleep. I had no idea where they came from or where they went. But there were opinions, chatter, judgments, planning, and statements that appeared factual but were later found to be blatantly false.

My mind was a never-ending source of mostly useless commentary on absolutely everything, re-creating a different past or planning the imaginary future, with the starring character in all of my stories being me.

Before I discovered mindfulness practices and meditation, I walked around most of the day in a trance, generally missing what was going on around me in real time because I was listening to these voices and inventing or replaying conversations in my mind. I could jog for an hour, listen to music, and incessantly think about past, future, and fantasy but had little memory of what I had seen on the run. I could have sex while thinking about what I was going to eat for dinner while simultaneously planning my appointments for the next day. I was completely absent from the present moment. And for about 45 years, I had no awareness that this was even happening. I was sleepwalking through my life.

While this sounds like the recollection of a psychotic person, this is the description of how the vast majority of us lives, being consumed with thoughts, listening to imaginary conversations, and spending only a fraction of our time being present. So what can we do about this seemingly normal state of the human condition?

> **Finally, I could understand why I said or did certain things and could start learning to care about all parts of myself, not just the likeable ones.**

Here's one really good option. It was my father who introduced me to "parts work," a system developed by psychologist Tom Holmes based on psychologist Richard Schwartz's work titled *Internal Family Systems* or IFS. While studying the role of members in family systems, it became clear that a single individual had personas within them that behaved in similar ways to members of a family system. Each of us, including the most psychologically aware and healthy, has several distinguishable personas within us that have vastly different capacities, opinions, and coping strategies.

Figuring this out, or at least starting to, using IFS principles is one of the most useful and deeply healing things I have ever done. Finally, I could understand why I said or did certain things and could start learning to care about all parts of myself, not just the likeable ones.

The Path from Misery to Happiness

After his death, I finally mustered the courage to read my father's book ti-tled *Steps to Happiness* by Taranatha, his Buddhist-given name. His path was described in beautiful detail, from being an alcoholic and a depressed physician with a miserable marriage, to finding peace and meaning as a Buddhist scholar and teacher. Not surprisingly, my first read involved flipping through the pages looking for my name and what my father said about me. Later, realizing that it wasn't all about me, I was able to sit down and really understand the path that this amazing man had made from misery to happiness.

My father described getting to know the various voices in his head. He invited them to speak and recognized that they all intended to be helpful despite their less-than-wise ways. He named them, loved them, and slowly gave the less helpful ones permission to slip into the background to allow his true Self to take the wheel. This concept amazed and enthralled me. I began to actively listen to who was talking in my head and getting to know their personas, quirks, and agendas. I gave them names, ages, and physical appearances. I use this in my coaching work with most clients, and it is incredibly helpful for almost everyone.

In a nutshell, here's how it works. The key is spending a significant amount of time sitting still, observing your thoughts—not climbing into bed with them but watching them as if you are a third person or a witness. Think of it like watching a movie on a screen but not jumping in to be an actor in the movie. You are a witness, not a participant. Journaling what you hear is helpful for discovering patterns. For most of us, the ability to do this is developed though contemplative practices. This doesn't mean you have to meditate for two hours a day for 20 years to get there. Meditating in quiet self-reflection or just sitting and observing your thoughts, if only for a few minutes, starts to give you the traction to look at your mind and its facets. Over time, whether days or maybe years, personas become clear. Then something magical happens. We realize that there is a watcher, an observer of all of this drama. Pure awareness. The Self.

For me, the personas were most apparent when I was triggered or in a highly emotional state. Whenever my speech or actions left me with a pit in my stomach, my body was telling me that one of my personas had come out to play. When I was not acting in alignment with my core values, my body would send a signal to stop. I'd feel sick, anxious, or like something was wrong. Once the craziness had passed, I was able to look back and ask myself who was doing the talking or acting. I could find patterns of behavior that eventually shook out into a handful of unique and different characters, each with her own opinions, wants, and fears. With more practice, I was able to shorten the duration of the limbic hijack and finally (sometimes) to circumvent it altogether by recognizing the voice of the persona in my head but not speaking or acting it out loud.

Most of us have a child, a critic, a manager or doer, a judge, and a people pleaser in their cast. There may be all types of other unique characters that represent parts of ourselves that got stuck at certain levels of development. According to the theory, amongst and often lost within all these personas is the true Self, who over time needs to be identified and developed as the primary driver of the bus with the ability to listen to the others but not act on their every whim. One of the key understandings is that all of these characters have good intentions, but due to their immaturity and lack of wisdom, they usually fall short of providing the most helpful advice.

You Can't Hate Them Away

If your inner critic, who is often one of the loudest of the crew, tells you not to try for that promotion because you're not smart, pretty, or skilled enough, her deepest intention is that you don't look foolish or fail. Understanding that she is trying to help, thanking her for her attempts, and then not surrendering to her advice is the key to allowing the true Self to be in control.

We cannot hate our personas out of existence, bury them, or pretend they aren't there. We have to hear what they have to say, understand their age, level of understanding and agenda, and that their purpose is to help us survive. Since these personas are stuck at various levels of development, some are very immature. Anyone throw a childish tantrum now and then? Some personas might be repeating the words of our critical caregivers. Once we fully know them and can meet them in the light, these "demons" become nothing more than rather unevolved friends. Consider the annoying relatives who give you unsolicited advice at Thanksgiving. You can listen with one ear, smile, and nod politely, but you don't have to believe or do what they say.

You may want these personas to go away, but they never will. They are part of you, and rather than being ignored, life gets a lot more peaceful and less confusing when you allow them all in. You can love them—you don't have to like them—and validate their opinions without giving them the car keys. Try having compassion for them and allowing them to be present but certainly don't let them be the primary decision-makers in your daily life. Remember, they are all doing the best that they can with their limited capacities.

> In my experience, deep genuine connection with another human can only exist if you are operating from your authentic Self.

A key concept here is *integration*, or putting all of these pieces together. Our common language somehow recognizes this reality when we say things like "pull yourself together" or describe someone as "falling apart," "going to pieces," or "Jekyll and Hyde." We seem to understand that we're comprised of many personas that ideally are integrated and working together with a hierarchy and control center that mirror Dan Siegel's fist model of the brain.

Bringing us back to the topic of this book, what does IFS have to do with sex and connection? In my experience, deep genuine connection with another human can only exist if you are operating from your authentic Self. If another inner someone—one of the damaged, immature ones—barges into the relationship, the connection is, by definition, inauthentic. When you find your true Self among the personas and learn how to keep her in the driver's seat in a healthy relationship with the rest of the characters, this allows you to really show up. From here, you can relate to others as your Self, unfettered by self-hate, judgment, fixed and immature views, and old conditioning. This is the person who can connect freely and intimately with a partner without shame, blame, or old stories and be free to experience the full potential of authentic lovemaking. She is already there, in you and in me. Yes, even us.

Meet the Cast

As an example of how this works, let me introduce you to some of my own cast of characters, and I hope you will have fun finding your own. In case you are wondering, doing this work doesn't mean that you're crazy.

It means you are actually sane enough to realize that we're all a bit crazy!

Suzle is the youngest member of the crew. Pronounced Soo-zil, which was my mother's diminutive name for me as a child, she's about five years old, terrified of abandonment, demands love and attention, throws fits, pouts, and understands things from a small child's perspective. It was Suzle who threw all of my wedding pictures out on the street and stomped on the frames during my divorce. As crazy as she can behave, Suzle's goal is literally to help me survive by not being abandoned. She just doesn't know how.

Madge, not coincidentally similar to my mother's name, is my inner critic, a grouchy old lady who reminds me to never say anything good about myself and never accept a compliment because I might get a big head. Madge believes it hurts much less to fall from a low place, so it's best to make myself inconspicuous. She's also the one who whispers, "Oh my, I can't believe she said that!" when I hear someone giving themselves a well-deserved compliment. Madge had me convinced for years that no one would ever read a book I wrote which is why I waited so long. Only later I was able to see that she was just trying to protect me from embarrassment.

Eyore is my inner persona who listens to Madge and agrees that I can never amount to anything, so I may as well give up. On those bad days when I lay in bed and can't get up, Eyore is in charge. During my divorce there were a lot of those days. Eyore was certain to remind me that I would always be alone, no one would want me, and my chances for happiness were over. Like Madge, Eyore thought that a preemptive strike at misery was better than being surprised. He's unwittingly trying to help.

Ironwoman has no time for any of these feelings and just gets the job done. She thinks all this psychobabble nonsense is bullshit. Ironwoman has been the leader of the crew throughout most of my life. She moved me to a different country at age 18 and got me through college (which I paid for by waiting tables), medical school, residency, and most of my first marriage. Ironwoman also helped me build a very successful business. She just wants to cut to the chase and avoid painful emotions and wasted time.

Malcolm X, one of my favorites, is an angry activist who gets furious about injustices, both real and perceived, and is always fighting for a cause. He is happy to rip off someone's head if they don't act in a caring, compassionate manner and creates enormous harm trying to make the world a better place. Malcolm X led angry peace protests when I was a teenager in the 1980s. Last year he fired my attorney for making a few real but (possibly) forgivable mistakes, leaving me without legal representation in the middle of an important dispute. As confused as he is in his delivery, Malcolm X really wants to make things better and is passionate about things being right and fair.

Candy is a newer member of the crew. She was identified by my coach Diana who noticed I often said things were okay when they clearly weren't. Candy represses all negative feelings and has sunshine and rainbows coming out of her head. She likes to show up when I meet new people and wants to appear positive and likable. Candy is an expert at spiritual bypass, which in a nutshell means operating as a spiritually advanced person who has it all together while completely ignoring the negative feelings that are still very much present. To well-trained observers like Diana, Candy appears less positive and more fake. Candy just wants everything to be okay and for everyone to be happy and to like her. Like the others, she means well.

Pab is a recently recognized cast member, and her name is an acronym for Passive Aggressive Bitch. I started by naming her Pam (for Passive Aggressive Mom) but realized she shows up in a lot of relationships, not just in my role as a mother. Pab says confusing things to my kids like, "Are you sure you want to wear that?" or "Just forget it! I'll put the dishes away myself!" In adult relationships, she might say something like, "Okay, so have a good time with your friends tonight! I guess I'll just go to a movie by myself." (That's an actual text I sent not too long ago. Yikes.) While studying how to be a more effective communicator with teens, I've learned to listen to Pab's annoying yacking and not have her words actually come out of my mouth. Sometimes Pab makes me start laughing for no reason now that I realize how ridiculous and unlikeable she is. When Pab wants to talk, I've found that silence is golden. No one likes her, particularly me. While it's hard for me to find the ways in which Pab is trying to help, I think she is just deathly afraid of honest conflict and wants to be appreciated.

Oprah is my primary operating persona and the one writing this book. Thanks, Oprah! Oprah is human and vulnerable with normal human feelings. She is not perfect, but she is patient, kind, strong, and self-aware. She can wrangle this crowd, listen to them intently with love on her interview couch, thank them politely, and then move forward with good decisions.

Tara is the last persona I've met so far. While she has no language, Tara is the silent and ever-present loving guide to Oprah. I can talk to Tara, but she doesn't answer with words. She is simply present and guides my actions by working through Oprah. When gut feelings tell me what to do, Tara is driving the bus. She just sits and waits silently, forever loving, compassionate, and never judgmental. Some would call Tara God. When I listen to her, through my body not through words, things usually go well.

Personas in Action

Personas have a silver lining. Sometimes, keeping less-than-helpful personas close by can be really useful. For example, in an emergency, Ironwoman can save a life or organize a team to put out a fire better than anyone. When my sister died in a car accident in rural Mexico and someone had to travel there to get her body back to the United States, Ironwoman flipped into action without pause or tears. If a patient or baby is in a critical emergency in the operating room, you want Ironwoman around. She is stone cold calm in critical situations. Malcolm X makes sure no one pulls anything over on me in a contract negotiation and prevents me from backing down when I'm acting for the greater good. Without his tenacity, I would not have been able to move my organization forward nearly as effectively because Malcolm X does not take no for an answer. Madge has probably saved me from genuinely harmful social embarrassment in the past. It's probably good that I didn't write this book until now and that I didn't start public speaking until my 40s because I didn't have much wisdom.

A client of mine is working on identifying his personas and recognizing how they interact with his partner's. *Shamu* is his inner child who grew up poor, overweight, and bullied by his classmates for living in a trailer park with an incredible young mom who worked two jobs to make ends meet. A key event in his childhood was getting a Shamu sweatshirt from SeaWorld. Having little else to wear that fit, he wore it most days. Shamu became obsessed with money, and anything to do with keeping or losing money became a trigger. Shamu is plagued with the belief that he is not good enough, does not have enough money or belongings, and that poverty and destitution are right around the corner.

A later-developing character we call *Meathead* joined the Air Force, lifted weights for hours a day, and developed Division I college talent in both baseball and football. He also had sex with countless women and got in bar fights with men who looked at him sideways. Meathead's aggression arose as an attempt to regain power and status from Shamu. When these guys get together with his partner's inner child, you can imagine what happens. It's like three adult-size first-graders trying to have a rational conversation. But amongst others he also has *Ajahn*, who is his highest Self. When Ajahn meets up with his partner's highest Self, the degree of love and connection is beyond this earth.

The point of all this work, and it's a lot of work, is to develop awareness about who is talking and what their agenda is. When Suzle (or Shamu) shows up, the most useful plan would be for the other to say, "I see you Suzle, and I love you, I accept you, you are welcome to be here, but we are not going to talk right now." Unfortunately, only the most highly trained individuals can master this because Suzle is so darn good at making you take the bait. These personas are really good at telling the same stories over and over, and they are highly convincing. Once you learn the patterns and the stories, you can recognize when they show up, identify which persona is talking, and see that this whole messy drama is actually a comedy.

It took me a long time to relate to my less likable personas with love. When I was first coached to take Suzle in my arms and give her the love she never received as a child, I thought, "God no. She's fat, ugly, horrible, and scary, and I don't want anything to do with her." Not only was my mother abandoning this child, I was abandoning her as well. Finding the soft, pure heart of this hurt child and loving her was the endpoint of years of very difficult work. I still can't stand her some of the time, but I forgive myself, and most importantly, I accept her. After all, she's just a scared little girl.

Christine also hears her critical voice as her mother:

> I went through this phase where I thought maybe I didn't deserve happiness. I would hear my mother in my head saying, 'This is what you need to settle for. He's a good man.' I would hear her voice saying, 'You need to stay with him. You won't find anyone better.' It was always her voice in my ear. The noise... the noise of

being taught you don't deserve the best... that you don't deserve to be happy... that your happiness is secondary. No, I had to give that up. I stopped listening to the noise. My happiness comes first, then when I'm happy, in turn the people around me can be happy.

Sometimes these crafty personas present as reality and speak to you in the first person. It takes a lot of work to figure out who's talking, but it can also be a lot of fun and is great practice for setting healthy boundaries. If you can't set boundaries with yourself, it's pretty hard to do it with anyone else.

At a recent meditation retreat, I was having a self-pitying moment and clearly heard a thought saying, "My life is a train wreck. How on earth can I give advice to other people when I can't even... blah blah blah." Before Eyore could finish his sentence, Oprah jumped in and cut him off firmly, responding, "That's NOT TRUE. And it's NOT KIND. I care about myself too much to let you speak to me that way." Way to go, Oprah! That entire interaction lasted just a few seconds and prevented me sitting for 45 minutes wallowing in self-hatred, pretending to meditate. If you had seen me sitting on that cushion, I had a faint smile on my face and adjusted my posture just a little straighter, silently high-fiving myself. Ahh. Inner peace is a journey, not a destination.

Dropping the Second Part

Inner critics are so ubiquitous and sneaky that they deserve a little more attention. A practice I invented and still personally work on daily to undo the harsh conditioning of the inner critic is called "dropping the second part." I have taught this to many clients and now even identify people who have a strong inner critic simply by listening for "the second part."

Here's how it works and a little history. About five years ago, one of my best friends and one of the only people who I can count on to tell me the truth gave me some brutally honest, constructive feedback. He told me that whenever I was in a conversation with him and getting to a place of connection, vulnerability, or intimacy, I would say something that ripped the carpet out from under him, leaving him feeling wounded. I was flabbergasted and wanted to understand more.

140 SEXUALLY WOKE

Here's how one of our conversations might have gone. "I'm really proud of myself for the seminar I gave today. I was really scared that it wouldn't go over well, but I think I reached a lot of people, and I got lots of good feedback," I'd proclaim. So far, so good. At this point, we were feeling really connected as friends and sharing a very nice moment. Then Madge would show up and scold in my ear, "You can't talk like that about yourself. How conceited and proud. Who do you think you are?" This chatter in my head sparked my dreaded "second part."

Here it comes. "But of course I'll never be as good at speaking as you. I just don't have that talent." To me, this seemed like a normal, self-effacing conversation. To my friend, I was taking back the connection we had established and then pulled away something precious that I had given him. To my friend it felt disconnecting, like I was stepping out of that soft place of vulnerability, as if I didn't trust him enough to stay in that shared space of intimacy.

The truth was I didn't trust myself to stay in that vulnerable space. "Much easier to fall from a lower branch," Madge would remind me. Here's the thing: Adding the second part is cowardly. Dropping it is brave and empowers you to climb up to a higher branch and stay there, despite feeling afraid.

A simpler version happens all the time when we get a compliment. "You look beautiful today. Those glasses really frame your face well," a friend might say. The appropriate and vulnerable answer is an appreciative thank you, not some version of the second part, such as, "These glasses? No, they aren't my favorites. They make my nose look huge." Crystal has her own version of this practice:

> I have trouble accepting things from others. I have had to work on that. It's even hard to accept a compliment. Someone told me my eyebrows look nice today. I think they're faded, and I want to get them tattooed. I don't like them at all. But you know what I said? 'Thank you. I appreciate that.' And I let it go. Now it's a habit to say, 'Thank you. I appreciate that,' and then just shut up. It's hard. No one wants to hear me say why they're wrong about my eyebrows because they're just trying to be nice.

This kind of thing really comes home to roost in a tenderhearted sexual relationship. Imagine a man with an utterly unguarded heart telling his 60-year-old beloved she's a beautiful woman. Then the beloved gives him the second part treatment. Ouch. Can you see how offensive that is to the person giving the compliment? Not only does it take the joy out of a potentially connecting moment, but it also gives back the gift of appreciation and doesn't allow the giver to benefit from the joy and merit of giving. Allowing others to be generous and kind is just the right thing to do. Sending back compliments is like refusing to accept a birthday gift you don't like. It's unkind and prevents connection.

> Sending back compliments is like refusing to accept a birthday gift you don't like. It's unkind and prevents connection.

Just Zip It

Listening to that inner critic and not accepting compliments is harmful to yourself and others. When I thought about it that way, I made it a daily practice to drop the second part. Just say the nice thing, or accept the nice thing, and then zip it.

When I first tried zipping it, I noticed how incredibly uncomfortable I was sitting in that space of silence. I literally almost had to bite my tongue. The ability to sit in a space of giving myself love without taking it back was almost unbearable. I would have to breathe, count, and tell myself, "Don't say it. Don't say it." Dropping the second part has gotten easier over time but still makes me uncomfortable. I would wait for the person I was speaking with to tell me I was vain and conceited, but no one ever did. They weren't Madge. They were real people with good hearts who genuinely wanted to connect with me. Boy, those inner critics are sticky and tricky.

One of my most memorable coaching clients came to me in her early-40s as a self-described 10/10 on the perfectionism, inner critic, and stress scale. Melissa, like many of my fast-paced executive clients, experienced a constant cycle of feeling inadequate because of the physical impossibility of being perfect at every aspect of her job. This led to constant worry and stress and elevated the volume of her ever-present inner critic's voice. That voice constantly told Melissa she wasn't good enough for her position, and if she didn't do a better job, someone would find out she was a fraud.

This cycle ran her life, and she worked way too much overtime. Melissa would go to the office on weekends to finish or double-check projects, leaving her husband and young sons to manage the house which was never clean enough when she got home. She was exhausted, and her sex life was non-existent. Through multiple sessions of coaching, Melissa was able to journal in the voice of her inner critic, who she named Ethel. She began to understand that Ethel was an old part of Melissa that mimicked her mother's voice, as inner critics often do, telling her she needed to work harder and be perfect to be accepted.

Melissa also became aware that in her own way, Ethel was trying to help Melissa succeed, albeit in a very cruel and ineffective way, and that she no longer needed to be obeyed. Melissa could hear Ethel's voice and answer softly but firmly, "No, thank you," from her authentic Self. Slowly, the cycle of a relentless quest toward unrealistic goals softened, Melissa's stress level diminished, her work hours returned to normal, and her relationship with her husband became much stronger and more connected. She made a practice of sitting in the driveway for two minutes to take relaxing breaths before entering the house. During those two minutes, Melissa also committed to connecting with her husband and kids for the evening, focusing on mindful listening, offering words of appreciation, and resisting the urge to launch into complaints about the state of the dishes.

> Listening to that inner critic and not accepting compliments is harmful to yourself and others. Just say the nice thing, or accept the nice thing, and then zip it.

Not surprisingly, their sex life returned and began to blossom. The dishes got done but oftentimes not until the next day. So what had changed? Melissa's workload, the state of her home, and the realities of having two young children were exactly the same. What changed is that Melissa was showing up as her true authentic Self. In her own words, "No one liked that other person. Everyone likes this one."

After a while, this process can become quite light and humorous. When Melissa now hears Ethel's critical voice, she can smile and say, "I see you Ethel, and I'm not falling for that old story again. I know you are trying to help, but it's not helpful; so please go, and sit down."

Unchained and Free

Many of my coaching clients and patients have had fun and experienced great growth and insight by doing this work. In the end, you can hear the persona talking, identify her, accept her with love, recognize her agenda, and not *believe what she's saying.*

Like my clients, I was freed from the tyranny and exhaustion of listening to unwise personas once I recognized that *they are not me,* rather they are just voices from parts of me that I created to protect me from an old or imaginary fear. With this realization I was able to see a clear path forward toward wisdom through Oprah and towards Tara. I could relax, be myself without shame, and have my mind and body in the same place. I could be present and connect with my body and my partner's, fully allowing whatever feelings arose to be there and to immerse myself in the experience from a position of freedom—which I define as not needing anything to be different. My integrated Self, loving all of my parts and personas but being clear about who is in the driver's seat, can experience the authenticity needed to connect genuinely without defenses and to love with an undefended heart. Can I do this all the time? Absolutely not! But being fully present and integrated even for a few minutes makes me know it's possible. And that means it's possible for you too.

Lovemaking with an undefended heart is a completely different animal than the sex with an agenda that we experience earlier in life. And it is almost entirely a deeply intimate and spiritual pleasure reserved for midlife. With few exceptions, if you work really hard, it takes about 40 or 50 years to figure this stuff out. Sadly most people never do. Perhaps some of you reading this will get a head start. I sure hope so.

EIGHT

Sexual Trauma and the #MeToo Era

B y now, the cat is out of the bag. Sexual violence against women is frighteningly common. More than 1 in 3 women interviewed for the MRS study had experienced rape or sexual assault. Keep in mind this was a group of women systematically chosen because they seemed to have the healthiest relationships with sex. Supporting national findings, most of these women never reported their rape or sexual assault to a counselor or anyone outside their families. Some of them never told anyone before me. Many of them were confused about whether they were somehow responsible or whether they accurately remembered what happened, often being wary about using terms like sexual assault or rape and even apologizing for their part in it.

We have been systematically trained to think no one will believe us. Maybe it didn't really even happen, and if it did, it was probably our fault. With this reality as the backdrop (even if we are not survivors ourselves but particularly if we are), how do we reconcile what has happened with what I am describing as potentially one of the most intimate and connecting acts of love that humans can experience? How can we open our hearts to complete vulnerability when we have been harmed so badly? How can we believe the universe is a benevolent place and trust that everyone is doing the best they can when we have experienced such cruelty and lack of compassion? And how can we live from a place of love, not fear, when our conditioning teaches us that fear is warranted? How do we open up to love when shutting down seems to provide the most reasonable means to improve our chance of survival? To answer these questions, we must first take an honest look at the problem, and then hear from the experts: women who have been through it.

Did That Really Happen?

I clearly remember my first confusing sexual experience when I was about six years old. In the early 1970s in New Zealand, nothing bad ever happened, at least that's what the prevalent thought process seemed to be. Kids walked alone to and from school every day, and parents just expected that we would show up at home in time for dinner. My elementary school was about half a mile from my house, and from the first day of first grade, the only way I ever got there was on foot.

One day as I was walking home alone as usual, a white pickup truck pulled up next to me. A man who I remember as being old—he was probably in his 50s—leaned over and rolled down the passenger-side window to talk to me. Polite, naive, and curious, I stopped. I remember his exact words because what he said was so strange. "Little girl, have you ever seen one of these?" As I looked in the window, I could see that his pants were down, and he was holding something that looked soft and furry in his hands. At first I thought it was a wrinkly baby chicken with fluffy light yellow hair. Another car approached, and the man drove away quickly. I continued home and never mentioned it to anyone. After all, I wasn't really sure what had happened. It wasn't until about five years later that I realized he was showing me his flaccid penis with a large puff of faded red pubic hair.

This can hardly count as sexual trauma. But it was certainly confusing and he was a pedophile who may have done much more serious things; so I was lucky. It's also an example of how crossing the line of what's appropriate and healthy in a sexual relationship can seem fuzzy, leaving us unsure about what happened and wondering if anything was really wrong. Rather than risk embarrassment or blame, we keep quiet. I shouldn't have stopped and talked to him. I knew better than that. If I told my parents, I likely would have been in trouble. And what would I have told them? A man with his pants down showed me a baby chicken?

At 14 when I *did* actually experience sexual trauma, I sure as heck didn't tell anyone. Everyone found out anyway, and guess who got in trouble? Only Charlene, as far as I knew. At that time in the early-80s, I didn't hear as much as a whisper about how those boys had done anything wrong, nor did I hear a whisper from myself. Even I believed it was all my fault, and not a mention was made of sexual assault, rape, or teaching these boys about a different way to approach girls and sexuality. It was just brushed under the rug. I truly believe that the adults who were aware of the situation blamed it entirely on the girls. Such was our conditioning. I believed it too. Even a few years later when my obsessively jealous boyfriend physically abused me, I never told anyone. I knew it was wrong, and I knew I needed to get away, but I was pretty certain no one would help me. I'm guessing I was right. At that time, no one talked about any of this stuff. It just silently happened to about 1 in 3 women, and that was just the way life was.

A little later when I was about 20 and living in Houston, my boyfriend James and I were sleeping off a big night of partying at his parents' house with a number of other young drunk bodies strewn about. I woke up at sunrise feeling someone's fingers inside my vagina. Half awake, I assumed it was James, so I let it go on for a minute until I was awake enough to realize it was really hurting. I sat up in bed and realized that one of my boyfriend's drunken friends had crawled in bed next to me. He apparently had been hiding under the bed planning his perverted attempt at courtship.

> My response illustrates how deeply rooted our acceptance of sexual assault was at that time and explains to me why the #MeToo Movement spread like wildfire.

My response illustrates how deeply rooted our acceptance of sexual assault was at that time and explains to me why the #MeToo Movement spread like wildfire. I mumbled sleepily something like, "What the hell are you doing??! Get the hell out of here!" James woke up, saw his friend, and they both started laughing. Then I started laughing. I don't know why except that it seemed to be the popular response. James asked his friend what he was doing, and the friend answered without shame, "I was just hiding under the bed; then I was fingering your girlfriend." Both broke out into uproarious laughter. It sounded like a funny line from *Beavis and Butthead,* and they repeated it in the appropriate voices. It was contagious. Apparently this was a hilarious event, and I didn't want to look uncool, so I went along.

After the rest of the house woke up, we all went out to a hangover-cure Mexican food breakfast. There were about a dozen people at the table, and the story of how James' friend had hidden under the bed waiting for me to be asleep so he could finger me was the source of great entertainment. We all thought it was really funny, even me and a handful of other girls. Tell anyone that I had been assaulted? Now *that* would have been funny. I didn't even consider it an assault until quite recently. After all, we were all drunk, I was passed out, and I shouldn't have been there in the first place. And boys will be boy—so I'd been told—and believed.

#MeToo, Too

When thousands of women came forward and told their stories of assault, abuse, and rape when the #MeToo Movement went viral in 2017, many of them had the same heartbreaking reason why they didn't speak up earlier. It must be hard to understand if you haven't experienced it, but many of us, just like me, weren't really sure if anything reportable had happened. The rest of the world seemed to think it was fine, so we just went along with it.

When high-profile sexual assault allegations began being widely publicized in 2016, so many of us wondered how this could happen—for example, how could an academically acclaimed professional woman my age be accused of lying about an attempted rape that happened when she was 15 when she had absolutely nothing to gain and everything to lose by coming forward? Although every piece of her testimony, including an FBI-administered polygraph test, pointed to her truthfulness, she was mocked and given the burden of proof to provide irrefutable evidence that a drunken teenage boy had abused her. When political leaders in the highest positions of our own government model this behavior and continue to hold their places in office, of course we won't come forward. The real statistics, I am guessing, are probably much more glaring than even the #MeToo Movement suggests.

This is not a book about the horrors of sex or a platform to debate politics. But understanding the shadow side of one of our most precious gifts is vital for those who have experienced trauma to move forward. We need to look at this head on so we can understand how to integrate our pasts into a future that does not allow trauma to define us or to define humanity.

Rosie, like many women, had a life-changing reaction to hearing other women's stories reported in the media. A strict Catholic, she was determined to wait until she was married to have sex:

> I had a serious boyfriend in college, and I was like, 'This is the real deal. I'm going to marry this guy.' Two months before graduation, my boyfriend was out of town, and I went to a party with some friends. We were all drinking. When the party was over, a boy I'd known since freshman year said he'd drive me home. I thought it was a safe idea. I knew this guy. So he drove me home, walked me upstairs... then he raped me.
>
> I went to an Ivy League school. There were a lot of rich, entitled boys. I remember him saying as he buckled his pants, 'No one will believe you if you make any trouble. My dad has lawyers. They'll make sure you don't have a life.' I had a feeling he had done this before. This was his M.O.
>
> Remember, this was the first time I'd ever had sex. I was drunk, but after he left, I had the sense to walk across the street to student health and told the nurse that I needed the morning-after pill. It was really strange. It was just such a normal thing for the nurse. She said, 'Okay, no problem.' I was expecting her to ask why, but she just went and got the pills and gave them to me. I thought, 'Wow, this must happen a lot. I guess I'm not going to make a big fuss about it.' And I was drunk. So it was my fault. It was like a box I just put all that into. I rationalized. This happens a lot. Girls have sex or get raped and threatened and then get the morning-after pill. This must be normal. What did I know?
>
> The problem was how I was going to tell my boyfriend. We had been waiting to do this together. I felt like I had reneged on my promise. I couldn't tell him. In fact, I never told anyone. So instead of telling the guy I was going to marry, I broke up with him. It was all I could think of to do. I just didn't want to have to ever explain this to him or anyone, so I just had to start over. That was in 1988. I didn't even go out on a date until 1991. I had the normal guilt our generation had about these things. Maybe I did something wrong, or I shouldn't have put myself in that situation.
>
> When this #MeToo thing was all over TV, I was watching women being attacked again, this time by the media, because

they couldn't remember the exact details of how it happened. I for one have no idea where the house was where we partied that night. I just remember it was big. I couldn't tell you what day it was. How can anyone be expected to remember that? Then it all came flooding back. I just broke down and cried. It was like I had to go through it all over again myself. I finally decided to tell someone, and I told my husband for the first time. I don't know what I had been afraid of. There was no blame or shame. We both cried, and he said, 'I'm just so sorry you had to go through that alone.'

I was at a reunion this year, and my girlfriends and I finally talked about it. Almost everyone had a similar story of being pinned down and molested or raped. I mean, it was almost everyone.

Dirty Little Secret

This is not about blaming the men and boys in these stories unless they intentionally lie about it afterwards (huh-hmm) because they were conditioned, the same way as us girls, to think that type of sexual violence was normal and even acceptable. As difficult as it is to swallow that a rapist or abuser is doing the best he can with what he's got in that moment, I still have to believe that it's true.

Sometimes the best a person has is just really, Really, REALLY poor and by no means does it let him off the hook. We are all 100 percent responsible for our actions. The perpetrators of these crimes did things and caused irreparable harm, and they are accountable for that for sure. But what surprised me the most in the recollection of my own experiences and through the stories from the MRS study was the degree of normalcy that existed around violence against women and how all of us, including both survivors and perpetrators, were conditioned to downplay or minimize it. It was one of society's dirty little secrets that no one really wanted to see. Almost everyone was involved in one way or another, even if only as a silent onlooker.

Maryann's story illustrates the almost unbelievable lack of recognition that sexual violence is wrong. She shares:

I think my relationship with sex was screwed up from the very beginning. I had no education around it at all. I went to an all-girls high school. I was very overweight. I had no interaction with boys. I never dated. When I was 18, I had nothing going for me. I graduated from high school in the mid-1970s and had no plans to do anything, so I moved to California where I had a relative.

I was walking down the block in my new city when I saw a guy cleaning his car. We started chatting, and after a while, he asked me out. I had never been asked out. Ever. I agreed, and we went to a drive-in and then back to his place. There he threatened to beat the shit out of me if I didn't submit. That's how I lost my virginity. When he was done, as I was pulling myself together to leave, he asked me out again! I guess it seemed like a normal date to him.

I didn't tell a soul. I didn't tell anyone for years. When all this #MeToo stuff blew up last year, I just had so much anger. I'm not an angry person, but I had just put this away ...stuffed it down for more than 35 years. Watching other women talk about going through this, I just couldn't believe this has happened to so many people.

No Means No

The last story I will share on this topic is about a different, less talked about form of sexual abuse that may be the last stone unturned in the #MeToo Movement: marital rape. Domestic violence of other sorts has received at least some recognition in modern society, and there are at least a few, albeit not nearly enough, resources for women who can produce bruises or broken bones to "prove" they're survivors of violence. But rape within a marriage is still viewed as a different animal. Very few legal systems even allowed for the prosecution of rape within marriage before the 1970s, and very few women will speak out about it since it's almost impossible to prove.

Denise recently divorced her husband of 25 years, whom she met when she was a teenager:

My marriage actually ended because of sex. I'm pretty sure my husband is a sex addict. It got worse and worse over the last few years. He would get more and more demanding, telling me to go down on him whenever he wanted and on his schedule. It was never enough. It had to be every day, sometimes more than once. When he wanted sex, he would look at me like food. I felt hunted. He would have a dead look in his eyes. He wasn't seeing me as a person anymore. He was seeing me as something to eat the same way he would look at a steak. When you see hunger in someone's eyes and they are physically much bigger than you, it's fucking terrifying.

He didn't care about my pleasure. He just demanded what he wanted and got angrier and angrier if I said I wasn't in the mood. We had really rough sex, and he needed to decide everything. He watched porn constantly. The worst night, he had sex with me against my will while I was crying. We talked about it afterward, and he said it wasn't the same as rape. I had so much anger toward him about that, but I would never tell anyone because I didn't want to hurt him or ruin his life. Plus after you get divorced, no one would believe you anyway. They would think I'm just trying to hurt him, and why is it just coming up now? What proof do I have? So I wonder by the same token how many thousands of women this is happening to because they will never speak up? No one will believe them. 99

Denise's chilling description of feeling hunted like food brings me back to the idea of animals and angels. While it's an oversimplification to say there are two kinds of sex, let's just assume for a moment that it's true. What Denise and other survivors of sexual assault experience is an extreme form of what I call "animal sex" or unevolved sex. Even animals can sometimes consent. And obviously "animal sex" between humans is usually consensual, as discussed earlier in this book, and can be plenty of self-centered fun when it's between two people who are each in it for what they can get for themselves. But this is about as far away from the sex of genuine love, generosity, and connection as you can get.

Shadows and Enemies

Carl Jung's brand of psychology recognizes a shadow in every person's consciousness. This language has been broadened in some spiritual traditions that recognize a shadow side or antithesis to every desirable emotion or action. In Buddhism, these are called "far enemies" or opposites. For example, the far enemy of love is hate (or ill will), and the far enemy of compassion is cruelty. Trickier, however, are the "near enemies" that can masquerade as their wholesome counterparts. For example, the near enemy of love is clinging or codependence, and the near enemy of compassion is pity. What these shadow sides and enemies have in common is that they are often confused with the real thing and one can turn into the other rather quickly.

It's hard to really understand without judgment how an innocent date can turn into rape and leave both parties confused, or how a husband can believe marriage grants him the right to treat his wife like property. But I think this understanding is vital if we're going to move away from the drama triangle with its victim, villain, and hero (the hero in this example might be the #MeToo Movement, an activist group, a political figure, me, or someone else) to a higher plain of consciousness that allows us to truly accept and be at peace with our pasts. Everyone did the best they could with what they were given at that moment. Breathe. Breathe. This is hard to read, I know, because it's hard to write. My Malcolm X would like to have all abusers hung up by the balls then castrated, but I'm pretty sure that wouldn't lead to peace.

> **It's an act of incredible bravery to open one's heart again after being seriously harmed.**

We need to forgive—not condone—and to separate sexual violence or even the more mundane varieties of disconnected sex from the possibility of real, loving, intimate sexual connection. They are two completely different things. If our only experience with sex is violent or disconnected, it's hard to imagine the world of possibility that we are missing. Until recently, I personally had no idea what I was missing. As long as we're the victim, we'll need a hero and a villain. But freedom lies on the other side of being identified by the trauma, stepping out of the drama triangle and seeing it for what it is: one big pile of pain and confusion where everyone loses. Forgive. Forgive yourself and everyone else involved, and you will find peace.

It's an act of incredible bravery to open one's heart again after being seriously harmed, and some of us never do. What's interesting is that each of the women I interviewed who had experienced sexual trauma *did* open their hearts again over time, and each of them found the love and genuine connection that had been so devastatingly absent in their earlier experience.

The pull toward love and light is mighty indeed, and nothing can stop it—not rape, war, abuse, or any shadow—if you are brave enough to follow that whisper from your highest Self who is patiently waiting to be born. To answer those questions posed at the start of this chapter, I will simply say *never give up*.

I am cautiously optimistic that we'll look back on this in 50 years with the same type of disbelief we now have about the Holocaust and slavery. Our children will read about this unfathomable time when women were treated as less than human and that sexual predators who lie and blame the survivors could be elected to the highest offices in the country. While the stories I heard in the MRS study occurred mostly in the 1970s and '80s, the problem has obviously not gone away, although I do believe the tide has begun to turn.

My teenagers, for example, cannot believe that we simply put up with men touching us inappropriately at work or making sexually inappropriate comments or that we didn't speak up about date rape or assault. It's hard for them to understand that it's the way life was back then and that in some ways not much has changed. But at least there's a conversation about it. They talk about it at high school, most of their peers seem to understand the concept of "no means no" (at least so far because they're 15 and 17) and that abusers are exposed, impeached, lose their jobs, or go to jail—and hopefully get educated and rehabilitated.

Like I said, I'm hopeful.

NINE

Sexuality and Physical Illness

J ust when we finally have the time, wisdom, and self-awareness to pursue the best sex of our lives, our bodies often have something else in mind. I'm pretty sure the original design of the human body was to die near age 50. In the modern day, many third-world countries still have a life expectancy in the 40s. From the 1500s until about 1800, life expectancy in Europe hovered somewhere in the 30s. Suffice it to say, even considering sex after 50 is a relatively new phenomenon.

Ironically, our ovaries—the part of our body that is the second most important, after our brain, for regulating our sexuality—get the message to "die" or cease functioning at around age 50 while the rest of our body lives on. With life expectancy for women in the United States now at 81, we can expect to spend a good 30-plus years post-menopause with good health and good luck.

We already talked about menopause-related anatomic changes and how those changes can do a number on your sex life. But the question remains: what are the other "complications" of aging that affect sex? And let's not forget that our male partners are getting older too.

Before we take all the blame, the incidence of erectile dysfunction (ED) increases from about 20 percent at age 40 to almost 50 percent by age 70. And with more than 3 million cases of prostate cancer in the United States every year, sexual dysfunction is the most common post-operative complaint. Heart disease, obesity, and diabetes can also contribute to ED, and the sharp rise in the use of antidepressants in "middle-aged" men and women, not to mention the rise of depression itself, is also a huge contributor to sexual dysfunction.

Thankfully, this isn't all bad news. A recurrent theme that warmed my heart in the interviews of the sexually woke was that the physical changes associated with aging often led to a radical shift toward an increase in connection. Watching our beloved partner suffer and struggle often seems to snap us out of the daydream we've been living in. It heightens our awareness that life is short and that every moment should be cherished. For me, the recent deep understanding that I will experience old age and death came not so much with a sense of despair or gloom but rather with an acute sense of the preciousness of life and the deep desire to savor every moment. I keep this quote framed on my office desk:

> *"Today I am fortunate to have woken up, I am alive,*
> *I have a precious human life, I am not going to waste it."*
> —His Holiness the Dalai Lama

Happiness Is an Inside Job

I'm extremely fortunate to have great health, and I'm still as active as ever and have no chronic health conditions. But sickness and death will happen. They happen to all of us.

So far, my one significant experience with a sex-life-altering health condition happened during the grueling 18-month child custody battle our family endured. It thankfully ended in my favor but not without significant psychological damage. While this chapter focuses on physical illness and not psychological illness, medical professionals are beginning to have a deeper understanding of the countless ways in which psychological stress can affect your physical body. Stress can kill you. Literally. Most of us know that heart attacks, high blood pressure, headaches, and stomach ulcers can be by-products of stress. Fewer of us know that stress and chronic high levels of stress hormones, including cortisol and adrenaline, can cause immune system dysfunction that can lead to pretty much every kind of physical illness, including cancer.

Fortunately, I didn't get cancer (this time), and thankfully my custody case didn't kill me or anyone else. But it came close. Despite years of mindfulness and meditation training and lots of professional help, I had some mental breaks that felt like I'd really lost it. My tears, insomnia, unsuccessful attempts to numb myself with alcohol, and wild mood swings resulted in some massive fights with those around me. The sheer insanity of being forced to endure and pay for a jury trial that we didn't ask for (only in Texas and maybe that will be the next book) frequently sent me to the guest room and even to a hotel and another country on several occasions.

At times it was emotionally unbearable, but that wasn't the worst of it. A trial of antidepressants to help with anxiety made me realize firsthand what I had been telling patients for years: antidepressants can kill your sex drive. Just when I needed to connect the most, one of my primary connection methods felt like it was going away. And it wasn't just the desire for sex that went away. It became almost impossible for me to have an orgasm. After trying and trying and trying—*whoosh*—the feeling would just disappear.

More than 10 percent of Americans take antidepressants, and the single largest group is women over 45, so it's safe to say that antidepressant use is a major cause of sexual dysfunction. However, the true effect is hard to measure since depression also causes a lack of libido in most people. So exactly how big a "thing" is it? We will never know. But trust me, it's big.

Antidepressants are also the most over-prescribed class of drugs in the Western world. In my practice, I'm confident that more than half of the patients taking antidepressants (prescribed by another doctor) have been misdiagnosed and are being mistreated. Depression and severe anxiety (the latter often also appropriately treated with certain antidepressants) can be life threatening and seriously debilitating conditions that can, no doubt, benefit tremendously from treatment. In fact, it's likely that antidepressants saved the lives of both my father and son. But being sad, worried, or stressed on occasion is part of normal human experience, particularly if something sad, worrisome, or stressful is happening.

Feeling our sometimes-unpleasant feelings is rarely a problem that needs to be treated with the exception of true major depression, severe and prolonged anxiety, or thoughts of self-harm. Instead, wait a while, exercise, meditate, talk to a friend or counselor, and change your lifestyle. In most cases, allowing the feelings to be present instead of stuffing or hiding them will allow them to pass through. There's no magic pill for happiness. If only it was that easy. You might have heard this before, but it's worth repeating:

"Happiness is an inside job." —William Arthur Ward

If you are on an antidepressant, really need to be on one, and are experiencing sexual side effects, here are some options. Exercise, counseling, and other lifestyle changes are just as important, if not more important, when you are being treated pharmacologically. One of my pet peeves is when doctors advise patients to "just take this pill" without adding any of the other non-medical treatments and without doing any work to get to the root cause of the problem. Doing so is just painting over rotten wood.

The most commonly prescribed class of antidepressants, called selective serotonin re-uptake inhibitors (SSRIs), is the worst culprit for sexual side effects. For many patients, drugs that work on a slightly different pathway, including dopamine or norepinephrine as well as serotonin, can work just as well without that miserable side effect. That was certainly the case for me. A short course of duloxetine (with the brand name Cymbalta) helped me sleep, kept the pendulum of mood swings from going too far in either direction, and allowed me to see that the future was still bright. And it didn't affect my sex drive. Phew!

Most importantly, get rid of the root cause if you can find it. If you cannot get rid of it, do some serious work to come to terms with and accept it, which is easier said than done. In my situation, my legal case ended in my favor. I felt like a new person within a week and accepted my new unplanned financial situation post-lawyers.

If only it was always that easy. And as always, check with your doctor—or find another one.

Not Always So

One of my favorite themes in life is that things we classify as "good" and "bad" aren't always so. Something might be unpleasant or pleasant temporarily, but to quote my teacher Vinny, "Just wait. It's not the end of the story."

Kimberly and her husband had been together for 40 years, but when Gary developed erectile dysfunction, they had trouble talking about it:

> Gary is a pretty healthy person, but he couldn't quite get an erection. Men don't really like to talk about that. I knew he had gone to see his doctor, but he was kind of secretive that day until I asked to see his paperwork for what was going on. The doctor had prescribed him one of those ED drugs, so we started talking about it, which was a big relief.
>
> We should have talked about it sooner. I think it's really getting to the depths of our vulnerability, the man's virility, strength, and ability to please and take care of us. I say that coming from a couple that's been together 40 years . . . It's amazing how difficult this was for us to talk about. I can't imagine if we had just met. Well, it was a huge relief for him to find out that he was okay, that ED is common with men his age, and that things can be done to help.
>
> The funny thing is I was just worried that I was not satisfying him. I never thought for a minute there was anything wrong with him, and all the while he's thinking that I was disappointed! We laughed a lot about that, and now it's like we're teenagers again. It's been really good for our relationship—the medicine and that it forced us to communicate and be open with each other. Who would have thought ED would turn into a good thing?

Carla has a similar story. Her father-in-law died of prostate cancer. Her husband John knew he was at increased risk, and he went to his doctor for regular screening tests. When John was in his early-50s, the blood test came back slightly high. "Nothing to worry about so far," she thought. To be on the safe side, John had a biopsy done, and they went to the doctor together to get the results. Carla remembers:

> The doctor said, 'Well, it's cancer, but you are lucky because we think it's really early.' The doctor went through the planned treatment, the high cure rate, and the possible side effects, but all I could think of was cancer. I could see John was getting really uncomfortable, and I was too. In my mind, I was thinking cancer. He might get really sick... and might die.

When we were in the car and after a long silence, he said, 'Are you going to be okay with this?' I told John I wasn't okay with him having cancer, but of course we would get through it. I ended my response with, 'What do you mean?' John reminded me that the doctor said, 'Our sex life might be different forever. He said he doesn't know. Maybe 50-50. Did you hear him?' I was like, 'Honey, if you are alive, that's all that matters.' Sex was the last thing I was thinking about, but it was the first thing John was thinking about. We had a good sex life, and for sure I would have missed that, but at that moment, it didn't matter. I knew we would be physically close whatever happened, and that would be just fine for me. We have this incredible bond, and I knew nothing would change that. All I thought was I just wanted John here.

I saw for the first time that for John, sex really defined him in some way. And I could see that fear, something primal that men have, that if he couldn't be a man in that way, I might leave him. John had the surgery, and we went to a post-operative visit with the nurse. She looked right at me and said, 'You have to give him six weeks, but then it's a use it or lose it situation. It's just like rehab. It's probably not going to be great a first but just keep trying.' I looked her straight in the eyes and said, 'No problem. I've got that covered.' During those six weeks, I read everything I could about how to ease back into things. Oral sex is best to start with as well as different things with the hands.

The funny thing is that right before that, our sex life had become a bit routine. We were just getting down to the business of it, and we had given up foreplay and touching each other slowly. So when we started trying at the six-week mark, I had to really listen to his body, take it slowly, and watch every response to see what was working and what wasn't. It was so beautiful in that way. We switched things around, so he would give me an orgasm first, either orally or manually like in the old days, and then I could focus on him. He already felt good about himself for making me feel good.

By about the six-month mark, we were able to have vaginal intercourse if he could get erect enough, but it didn't matter so much if there was an end point. He already felt good because he was pleasing me. I joked with him, 'The shoe's on the other foot now, buddy!' because I would have to be so in tune with his breathing and the release in his body to know when he had an orgasm since there was no sperm. I'd tease, 'Now I have to wonder if YOU are faking it!'

I wouldn't suggest that everyone's husband get prostate cancer, but for us, it's been awesome in many ways. First, after surgery I was always the initiator. I would remind him the nurse said to use it or lose it, that it was physical therapy . . . Let's do this! That really stroked his ego. The best thing is it caused us to just slow down and completely reinvent what was probably going to die a slow death if we had kept going in a monotonous direction. We had stopped really paying attention to each other's bodies in that really present way. So it's weird to say, but sex is now better than ever in many ways.

Daniella had another story of how this phenomenon works when faced with an unexpected illness. You might recall that she and Carl had always had a really healthy sex life that was an integral part of their lives. Then something hit them from out of the blue:

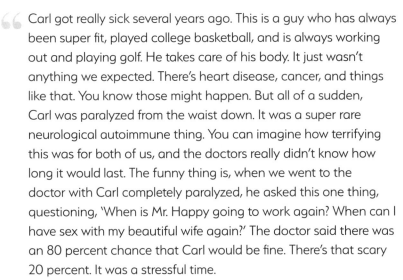

Carl got really sick several years ago. This is a guy who has always been super fit, played college basketball, and is always working out and playing golf. He takes care of his body. It just wasn't anything we expected. There's heart disease, cancer, and things like that. You know those might happen. But all of a sudden, Carl was paralyzed from the waist down. It was a super rare neurological autoimmune thing. You can imagine how terrifying this was for both of us, and the doctors really didn't know how long it would last. The funny thing is, when we went to the doctor with Carl completely paralyzed, he asked this one thing, questioning, 'When is Mr. Happy going to work again? When can I have sex with my beautiful wife again?' The doctor said there was an 80 percent chance that Carl would be fine. There's that scary 20 percent. It was a stressful time.

Thankfully, Carl fell into the 80 percent, and he is sexually fine now, but for several months we just didn't know. He's playing golf, walking, and doing normal things again. Now I see him slowing down a bit. Carl doesn't have the stamina he used to, and I am starting to see the old man I'm going to care for. In a way, it's tested our love, and I love him even more. Carl never lost his sense of humor. The good part about that horrible episode is that it really put a little jump in our step. We have always been in love, but after this, we just appreciate each other even more. We know life can change like that. You never know when it will change, and we'd better enjoy each other every minute. 99

The Dreaded News

While we will all get sick and die from one thing or another, few illnesses are closer to most of our hearts than breast cancer. With 1 in 8 American women now developing breast cancer in our lifetimes, it's something I've pretty much resigned myself to being diagnosed with at some point. Every time I get my mammogram, I'm ready.

Cancer specialists who focus on the single metric of a cure for cancer are proud to report that the great majority of early breast cancers are completely curable, and survivors can expect a normal life expectancy. The problem with this great news is that it completely fails to take into account the devastating effect it can have on intimacy.

Common treatments typically wipe out your two biggest sex organs (besides the brain): breasts and ovaries. Surgery can leave your chest numb and disfigured. Medical treatment can throw you into menopause overnight if you're not there already, and you can't take estrogen to help with the symptoms. It can feel like a complete nightmare during a time that you're expected to be celebrating your good fortune for being cancer free.

Shari was diagnosed with breast cancer at 45, which should not have been a huge surprise in light of her family history. Still it was devastating news. With three girls all shy of high school and a big job that primarily supported the family, Shari didn't have time to be sick, and dying wasn't an option. Even though the cancer was early-stage, she opted for a bilateral mastectomy due to her genetic and family history. She also had her uterus and ovaries removed:

66 When I was discussing all this with my doctors, it seemed like an easy decision. 'Let's just get this shit over with,' I told her. 'If my chance of ovarian cancer is high and if I'm going to be in menopause with the medicine anyway, just take it all out. And I'm not going to get a mammogram every year waiting for it to come

back. Just take both of them off too.' Of course, I was talking to cancer doctors, and I had the best ones at M.D. Anderson Cancer Center in Houston. I felt lucky. I would be cured, and then I could get back to work, and everything would be hunky dory.

The doctors were truly amazing, and they saved my life, but understandably all they cared about was getting rid of cancer. They weren't too concerned about what else might happen after the surgery. I don't think I would have made a different decision if I had known how hard this would make other aspects of my life, but I certainly would have thought harder about it. The surgery was a bear, but it all went well, and I healed fine. I had a kind of tummy tuck to get tissue to make new breasts. In clothes, I look normal— better even. But naked, I feel like Frankenstein. I have so many scars. My breasts are mounds that are in about the right place, but they are totally numb, and my tummy... well, let's just say I won't be wearing a bikini ever again. That all might sound vain, but when you don't want to be seen naked and can't feel anything, romance is not at the top of your list.

The worst part was the menopause. I had no idea. I should have asked more about that. Most women go through it over a few years, but I went through it in one day. WHAM! I had every symptom under the sun. Hot flashes, night sweats, mood swings, insomnia... the works. I felt so depressed. My doctor thought I was grieving about having cancer, but I assured her, 'I don't have cancer. I have menopause. I just feel like crap!' After the surgery, we weren't allowed to have sex for six weeks anyway, but we gave it a valiant effort once we got the green light. It took a while to admit it, but I couldn't feel anything except pain. My vagina was so dry we had to use lubricant, and even then I felt like I was being stabbed with a knife, and there was no way I could have an orgasm unless we pulled out all the stops. I mean it was work. The energy it took to try to be how we were before was just exhausting.

I'm not sure how we got to this point exactly, but now almost three years later, we are just really at peace with this new life we have. The cancer changed everything, but hey, I'm alive. The hot flashes and other symptoms, except the vaginal dryness, finally subsided. We don't have vaginal intercourse anymore, like ever. It just hurts too much, but we are both really okay with that. To tell you the truth, I always preferred oral sex anyway. I can feel good with that and have an orgasm some of the time. He likes oral sex, too, so we can still be really close. We are happy with that. I'm less conscious about my weird-looking naked body, and hey, we all look a little weird as we get older. I think I just woke up one day and said to myself, 'I have two choices here. Either keep fighting reality and be exhausted, or create something new out of this that can be good.' Everything changes. This is just a new phase. "

The Power of the Uterus

Having a hysterectomy, even when you're well beyond needing it for childbearing, often comes with a rush of emotion and attachment. More than just a vessel to hold a baby, many women associate the uterus with their femininity and womanhood. I've had patients ask, "Will I still be a full woman if I don't have a uterus?" Many women wonder if sex will be affected, if they will still be able to have an orgasm, and if their partner will notice anything. The answer to those questions is no—except maybe positively since your original problem will be cured—absolutely yes, and not at all. I can talk until I'm blue in the face about the scientific reality that the uterus is about as useless as the appendix when you're not wanting more children, but it's been helpful to use more empathetic language. Personally, I would happily hand my uterus over if there was a good reason to take it out, but to some people, it's a big deal.

Reverend Linda has an interesting take on her own surgery:

" Having a hysterectomy was in many ways deeply liberating. Not only was I cured of the problem that required surgery, but it was more than that. Losing my uterus was an invitation to think about being a woman in a different way. The uterus has the energy of being mother, symbolic woman, God woman and all that. In the role of mother or church leader, some female priests in my tradition even go by 'mother.' I have never been one of those priests, but your energy can get drawn out that way. Now I can care for people without that symbolic title. It feels more free. I moved from mother to person. It's almost as if there are more places I can go with that. "

Peace

The point of this chapter isn't to make light of serious illnesses and suggest that everything will always turn out fine, although my research was pretty clear that it oftentimes does. Things change, and suffering is real, but something about the acceptance of our new aging and physically changing state (or that of our partner) comes with a real sense of peace. That's my greatest wish for each of us as we go through this together.

TEN

Sex and Self-Worth

The feeling that *I am not good enough or that something is wrong with me*, might be the most common and pervasive feeling that humans share, particularly women in the Western world. My mother was taught this and passed it on to me, and our capitalist society largely depends on it continuing. We all know this on some level, but if everyone was content and felt good about themselves, our economy as we know it would implode. We'd stop constantly buying things in a hopeless attempt to make ourselves happy.

There's a potential problem with all books in the self-help genre. At its essence, this book is hoping to point to a "better" way of being. This is a perfect setup for assuming something is wrong in the first place. It's a slippery slope. So let me start this discussion of self-worth by suggesting that *nothing is wrong with any of us*, but we all have some harmful conditioning to undo to grow into our greatest potential.

Fact and Story

Harmful conditioning comes in many forms. Consciously or not, we have absorbed many, many years of teaching from our caretakers, schools, churches, past relationships, the media, and genetic programming. From my own experience and that of my patients, I can confidently say that almost all of the teachings we commonly receive about menopause and sexuality do not enhance well-being. They are also flat-out *not true*. Let me give you some examples. Women over 50 are not sexy. All wrinkles need to be eliminated. Thin people don't have cellulite. Our bodies should always look the way they did when we were 20. Men prefer younger women. Being attractive after 50 requires plastic surgery. Trying new sexual activities is dirty or wrong. There's no reason to have a sex drive when you're done having babies. The vagina inevitably dries up after menopause. Gray hair is unacceptable. Older gay women are lonely and surrounded by cats. Think how many of your own teachings you might have to add to that list.

I have an exercise called "fact and story" that we do at my office adapted from the Conscious Leadership Group. The gist is that we're encouraged to explain a situation using just irrefutable, unarguable facts. We do it a second time using a bunch of assumptions, opinions, and drama. The latter is always really funny and makes us acutely aware that most of what we think and say is a story. For sure, most of it is arguable or refutable. The last step of the game is to challenge our ideas and assumptions by imagining that the opposite of our story is at least as true. Why not, if it's actually just a story? For example, what if women over *50 could be sexy*? What if the vagina *might not* inevitably dry up after menopause? What if trying new sexual activities *possibly isn't* dirty or wrong? What if older gay women *can* be perfectly happy, thank you.

> Almost all of the teachings we commonly receive about menopause and sexuality do not enhance well-being. They are also flat-out not true.

While you're wrapping your mind around that, let's think about earlier conditioning that we may have received and incorporated into our collective view of what's true. It was my fault that he mistreated me. I deserved to be treated badly. There's no point in trying because things never work out for me. Boys will be boys. That's just the way men are. People are not trustworthy and always leave. Something about me is unlovable. *Something is wrong with me.*

Challenging our age-old assumptions is really, well—challenging. Realizing that some of our core beliefs are just stories can feel like losing a best friend. Sure, she may have been a really harmful and critical best friend, but she was reliable.

Breaking the Chain

Crystal shared how early conditioning showed up in her life, how she took the incredibly brave step to challenge her assumptions, and how she has created a healthier path. Remember, her first sexual experience was being molested by her stepfather, and to this day, her mother has never acknowledged the immense pain of Crystal's childhood by instead recalling that everything was "just fine." She shares:

> My mother's brother and I were talking a while back when she was sick. I asked my uncle, 'Why does she always see things with rose-colored glasses? What happened to her growing up?' He told me that when my mother was 18, she went to a party. She flirted with three soldiers who he said thought she was cute because she was light skinned. My uncle said with a weirdly accusatory tone, 'And they raped her.' I immediately snapped back, 'I don't care how cute a woman thinks she is; that gives no man a right to rape her! I know I'm beautiful, but that does not mean that someone has the right to assault me!'
>
> I did the math, and this was in 1954. In those days, if a woman flirted and was assaulted, then the crime was the fault of the woman. Women were shamed and told that they were less of a person, particularly women who were black. My uncle and my mom were raised to believe that.
>
> It explains so much about how I grew up. My mother did not tell me about my period. We did not discuss sex in our household. She did not tell me that no one should touch me without my permission. And after child protection services visited the house, she did not discuss that her new husband was sexually molesting me. When we became adults, my younger sister told me he was molesting her also. We have to break the chain to save our daughters.

Buying in to the story that "I deserve this, and I am not worth better" is pretty understandable if that's all that you are taught. But at some point, like Crystal, we are responsible for challenging our own assumptions and calling BS on those old stories. Crystal continues:

> I used to have this deep, dark hole in the center of my heart, which I blamed on the abuse I endured as a child. Not being in control and being exposed to sex at a young age damaged me. I was a victim. As such, I felt like I had no control.
>
> As a young adult, I used sex as a way to show myself that I was in control. I learned what I like and what I don't enjoy at all. It took so much therapy to help me realize that I don't want just sex. What I also want is someone to listen to me, love me unconditionally, and work alongside me to help me reach my goals. A true partner is what I crave. I don't need my husband, but I want him in my life. We enjoy being around one another. I had to grow up and acknowledge what happened to me as a child and use it as a stepping-stone, not as an excuse to not become someone amazing. I had to stop being a victim.
>
> Now I focus on breaking the chain and teaching the younger women behind me what they are capable of doing. Men are expected to enjoy sex. Women are shamed for enjoying it. But women are just as human as men. We deserve to enjoy and love our bodies just as much as men enjoy and love theirs. If a man can stand in front of the mirror, rub his belly, and still think he's so hot, well, then so can I!

Hearing this account of one brave woman, we can see how many limiting and harmful assumptions she challenged and changed. Crystal had every excuse to stay in the victim role and complain about all the ways life had treated her unjustly. Harmful parenting, abuse, neglect, and racism all could have defined her. If she had allowed herself to be defined this way, Crystal would have validated the story that she was "less than" and not worthy of love and happiness.

Self-Compassion or Self-Esteem

Here's one of the most important things I have ever learned: *in as much as we believe any form of diminished self-worth, I promise you, we are believing a story that is not true*. Each of us is inherently perfect and has equal worth. It's only the stuff we pile on to hide our true nature that makes us appear any form of "less than." Whatever your religion or belief system, I hope this can resonate with you.

As Reverend Linda beautifully explained to me, "The image of God is in everyone. Maybe we forgot it or lost it or actively deny it, but it's there in everybody." Everybody. That means you and me. If you don't use the word "god," change it to a word that makes sense to you.

Kimberly remarks:

> God loves us more than anything. He loves me just as much as some seemingly crummy person. I mean, some people have done some really awful things, but He still loves them like He loves me. It helped me to realize that and be aware that I am special, but I'm not more special than that person. Our greatest goal is to love one another and treat each other with respect. So I need to treat myself that way too. Why am I the only person in the world not worthy of love? I'm not that special. We are all loved by God.

Believing this at a heart level can butt up against a lifetime of conditioning that I'm a second-class citizen in some way, and it takes A LOT of practice to constantly remind myself that I am as lovable as anyone. Ironically, the modern focus on building self-esteem has definitely backfired and caused serious downsides. The problem with the self-esteem movement is that it encourages us to feel special and above average to feel okay. Calling someone "average" is an insult. But guess what? Statistically speaking, the great majority of us hover close to average in every way. That's what average means! Pursuing high self-esteem has a divisive component because it's based on being better than someone else. There is a comparison element that can cause enormous pain. Basically it's an exercise in Ego building that can lead to aggression, prejudice, and anger.

Building a sense of self-worth and self-compassion is very different and may just seem like semantics, but to me it's really an important shift. I have been fortunate to attend several seminars led by self-compassion author and researcher Dr. Kristin Neff, and I think her work should be required reading for being human:

> **Pursuing high self-esteem has a divisive component because it's based on being better than someone else. There is a comparison element that can cause enormous pain.**

"It's important to distinguish self-compassion from self-esteem. Self-esteem refers to the degree to which we evaluate ourselves positively. It represents how much we like or value ourselves and is often based on comparisons with others. In contrast, self-compassion is not based on positive judgments or evaluations; it is a way of relating to ourselves. People feel self-compassion because they are human beings, not because they are special or above average. It emphasizes interconnectedness rather than separateness. That means that with self-compassion, you don't have to feel better than others to feel good about yourself. It also offers more emotional stability than self-esteem because it's always there for you—when you're on top of the world or flat on your face."
—Dr. Kristin Neff

How we feel about ourselves in this way and how willing we are to offer ourselves compassion plays out mightily in romantic and sexual relationships. The great majority of women in midlife were taught some version of what I learned: loving yourself is selfish and proud, and the appropriate response to your own pain is to beat yourself with a shame stick. From this self-flagellating and apologetic position, you become a perfect target for subtle and outright abuse because in some way you believe that you deserve it. This misunderstanding plays out in imbalanced relationships with one person having power over the other (most frequently the male over the female). Something in the back of your mind tells you to be nice, pretty, and polite. Don't offend anyone. Take whatever is given to you. In this pool of confusion, it's impossible to build a truly connected and balanced relationship. In Robin's words:

> If you're in that place where you've excluded yourself from love and compassion, to me it seems impossible to have a connected, intimate relationship. You're just sort of showing up as half of a person. There was so much of myself that I shut off. I wasn't able to be seen.

Veronica says it in a different but similar way:

> I felt this way when I was younger: sex was a duty. As a woman, as a wife, it's our duty. What we want doesn't matter. That's when

you get into those binds and chains, and you're not free anymore. There's no balance. Been there, done that. It's horrible. But you don't quite know what else to do. A lot of women with a very strong faith are stuck in that misunderstanding. But once we are in a fully connected relationship with an equal power balance, that's when we can really connect, be it sexually or whatever. If we're not in balance and someone has the power and someone else doesn't, how can we be really connected? That's an employer/ employee relationship. It's not balanced.

No one is to blame for this situation—remember that we are all doing the best we can with what we are at this moment—but we each have to take responsibly to change it, both men and women, if we're going to move toward awakening, including sexual awakening.

Maryann describes:

All my life I've had to deal with that male "gaze" that sees me not as a person but as an object for their satisfaction. I think women often look at men that way, too, like you are here to make me happy; you are here to complete me. This is such a selfish, self-centered view. I would tell men all my life, 'Don't you get it? I'm just like you. Whatever is happening internally to you about your hopes, dreams, and fears, that is all happening to me too.' They would say, 'Of course, I know that,' but they didn't really get it. They would be talking about women this and women that like, 'Can't live with them; can't live without them.' What the F? And I hear some women saying those things too.

I think it's so interesting and hard for us that there's this construct that we're all free and doing our autonomous individual thing, but that is total BS. Our cultural narrative of freedom is overlaid with the reality that we are still second-class citizens. Culturally we've been taught to be a sort of second-rate person because we are female. Our expectations of one another as men and women are still in very narrowly constrained and confined roles.

I think this is really true. Granted, we have come a long way. We can vote, have access to education, can run for president, and have new freedoms in many ways, at least in the West. But we are still far from equal, even in most of our own minds.

One of my favorite stories from my interviews came from Christine as she talked about her teenage son and his first date. Her complete honesty really made me stop and think:

> My son asked my husband, 'Can I buy flowers for my girlfriend like you do for mom?' My husband said, 'If you wash the car, sure, I'll buy you some flowers for your girlfriend.' So the day came for the date, and I was talking to the girl's mother about the flowers. Something struck me as odd. The mother said worriedly, 'If they break up, she is going to be spoiled and think all guys are supposed to treat her that way.'
>
> I said, 'Well she's your daughter. Shouldn't you teach her that all guys are supposed to treat her that way?' Here we are raising another generation of girls thinking they are not good enough. Oh my gosh, can we just break the cycle? That's what I would tell other women. Set the example for your daughters. 'No, you will not treat me that way.' If we don't, there's going to be another generation of women being mistreated, not sexually satisfied, and just not living to their best potential. Don't do that.
>
> I went out recently with a girlfriend who had just gotten divorced. Her husband left her for someone younger. My friend said, 'What am I going to do? The guys are terrible. They all cheat.' I said, 'That's because we have a generation of women that's allowing them to be terrible. You need to demand what you want. Demand what you deserve. You're not being unreasonable.' She replied, 'But then they will just go with someone who will put up with that.'
>
> See, that's the issue. If we all got together and said, 'I'm worth it. I will not be treated like that,' then maybe we wouldn't have this problem. I'm not blaming women, but to be honest, we have to take our share of responsibility. Maybe 'insist' is a better word than 'demand.' But then that goes right back to women apologizing; we don't deserve to 'demand.' Maybe it would be nicer if I just 'insisted.' I hear the word 'demand,' and I'm like, 'Wait a minute,

I can't say that.' It's so deeply ingrained. We are taught that it's arrogant to ask for what you want. But in a way, isn't it arrogant to think you are especially NOT worthy of what you want? We have a lot of work to do.

You Can't Give What You Don't Have

Yes, we have a lot of work to do on ourselves, and until we have done that work, it will be really difficult to set a good example for our daughters and sons. I almost hate to repeat the overused bumper sticker cliché "You can't love someone else until you love yourself." But let's face it, a lot of clichés are true. I really didn't understand what that meant until recently. Lots of people talk the talk but don't or can't walk the walk. Whitney Houston sang about it (we all remember "Greatest Love of All") and tragically died from a drug overdose after years of addiction and self-hate.

What that statement means to me is that you can't give from a place of scarcity. You can't give what you don't have. You might feel like you love someone, but from a scarcity mentality, it's a love based on the need to fill something missing in yourself. Until you love yourself and don't have any holes to fill, relationships—even with our children—will have an element of clinging or needing which is based in fear, not love.

As a recovering codependent I would have argued loudly about that statement until quite recently. After all, I deeply loved my kids, my family, my patients, and my work. But in retrospect it was a love based on the need to be lovable. All of my relationships were set up to prove to myself that I was worthy of love because I didn't love myself. After every achievement I would silently ask the world "Am I lovable now? Am I lovable now?" But I got no answer from the outside, so I kept trying. I tried so, so hard, never knowing that just by being still I could find that love from within myself.

We have to break this cycle and show our children a better way. Christine adds a great perspective about setting a good example:

I want my kids to see that my husband and I are affectionate toward each other. I don't want them to end up in a relationship where they think it's okay to not be affectionate and not love each other. They deserve that. I deserve that. I want us to give them that example. You deserve someone to cuddle you and tell you, 'It's okay; I'm here with you. I want you to feel like you are at home. You are worthy of love. You are worthy to be hugged and kissed and touched.' 🙶

There are so many layers in the trance of unworthiness, that "I'm not good enough because I don't meet the standard." There are so many potholes to fall into when your sense of self is so fragile and dependent on others. Your sense of self is unreliable. When it comes down to it, no one but yourself can be ultimately reliable. *You are the only one who is guaranteed to be with you until the end, through thick and thin.* If you are in this unworthy state—I'm not good enough. My stomach is sticking out. My skin is saggy. I have cellulite. I'm worried about my hair—how can you be free to be yourself in a loving relationship? And how can you support yourself no matter what happens?

If we feel unworthy, we won't show up fully for fear of being seen as unworthy, and we will cling to compliments or being told that we are okay by someone else. We almost don't exist without validation from outside. Unless this changes, we live in a precarious and dependent position. Our happiness is dependent on others. That never, ever works.

Robin continues:

🙶 You don't believe you're good enough, so you put up with mistreatment. You want the lights out, eyes closed, and in your nightie or a robe. You're not able to really participate in a sexual relationship or the family as a whole person. You can't be your whole, free self if you're worried about how you look or comparing yourself to some ridiculous standard. So you check out and just go along in a dream. It's like counting the days. One day it will be better. One day. But you know what? That day never comes unless you wake up. I had to wake up. That day is today, or it's never. I'm not living that way anymore.

A lot of us grow up with so much of a mismatch of what we are told about sex compared with the real beautiful potential of sex. People are kind of hung up on the dirtiness or not wanting to let go and fully participate because they feel like it is unholy or whatever. I think their understanding isn't fully formed. If you have a fully formed spiritual understanding when you are in a true partnership, then that can be the grounds through which you connect with God or the universe in a way. In connecting with your partner as an equal, giving and receiving unconditional love, you can see that we are all really connected and lovable, one person at a time.

Sex and Privilege

This unworthiness disease plays out in an even louder way for women in racial and sexual minorities. In a marginalized group, you are often forced to struggle with feeling good enough every day while society constantly barrages you with information suggesting that you are not. As a heterosexual white woman, I have enormous privilege based on those two facts alone. It's impossible for me to truly understand what it feels like to be otherwise. With enormous gratitude, some of my interviews provided a window into the world where so many women live. As a biracial woman, Crystal describes:

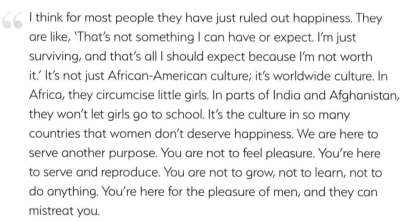

I think for most people they have just ruled out happiness. They are like, 'That's not something I can have or expect. I'm just surviving, and that's all I should expect because I'm not worth it.' It's not just African-American culture; it's worldwide culture. In Africa, they circumcise little girls. In parts of India and Afghanistan, they won't let girls go to school. It's the culture in so many countries that women don't deserve happiness. We are here to serve another purpose. You are not to feel pleasure. You're here to serve and reproduce. You are not to grow, not to learn, not to do anything. You're here for the pleasure of men, and they can mistreat you.

And there is a certain way you should look. I am the product of two biracial parents. My hair is super, super curly. I used to flatiron my hair because I was told, 'This is what's sexy.' I would plan my workouts around my hair. When I had sex, I had to be on top so I didn't mess it up. I'm done with that now. I mean, it was exhausting. Now I'm like, 'This is my hair. Take it, or leave it.'

Alexa gives a great perspective as a bisexual woman:

> I think we have some ingrained sense of 'I'm not good enough. I cannot do this. Any little mistake means I'm unqualified.' People can fall into this trap of thinking 'I'm not good enough, so someone needs to fill up this black hole inside of me.' But nothing good comes from that. For me, I identify as being bisexual, and when I was younger, I was gay. That's a kind of catastrophic way of not being good enough which can crush somebody's spirit. It can be so catastrophic that I think some sexual minority people say at some point, 'Wait a minute. The game is rigged. Being who I am, there's no chance in hell that I will be what society says I should be. So I'm just going to do my own thing.'
>
> I always thought I was a failed horse until I went to Berkeley, where I found out I was a zebra on a campus with lots of other zebras!
>
> That can be the powerful upside. You can't change the color of your skin, and you can't change your sexuality, so you might as well give yourself a pass and just live your life. There's a fork in the road, and you can choose to keep on that hamster wheel trying harder and harder to fit in, or you can just jump off and be yourself. There's something potentially liberating in that.
>
> Carl Jung was famous for saying that in the second half of life, people's values can change. We can become more at home with who we are. Or maybe we can find each other and say, 'Let's be at home with who we are together.'

While I don't know what it's like to be in a sexual or racial minority, I do know what it's like to experience ageism, mainly coming from myself. I am constantly catching myself judging myself for being in my early-50s. Elizabeth can relate to that feeling:

> A lot of people, for whatever reason, give up. There's the underlying feeling, this pervasive feeling that we are not worth it; I'm old now so what's the point. The way I look at it, we're going to live until 85 or 90. That's a long time left to live if you give up at 50. That seems like why bother even leaving the house? Why bother taking care of myself and staying engaged in life? Why

bother doing anything? I think it's because society is saying, 'Well, you are that age now. You are in menopause. That's just the way things are.' I know a lot of women like that. It takes energy to move forward and challenge that idea. 99

I'll end this chapter with an idea vocalized by Denise:

66 When you think about the story of your life until now, most of us were very reactive. I would like to learn to be proactive and recognize my own needs. I don't need to wait for a man to need me. I'm now in the dating world again after my divorce, and I feel myself waiting for him to take the first step. Why can't I just say, 'Hey, I'd like to have sex,' if that's how I'm feeling? We are taught to wait. We are not supposed to ask. We are not supposed to listen to our own bodies and take care of our own needs. I hope that changes. 99

I hope that changes too. We have thousands of years of conditioning to undo to stop believing on some level that we are second-class citizens. First, we need to believe it ourselves. We can blame men, our parents, or teachers for keeping us in this state of unworthiness, but as long as we believe it ourselves, we are stuck.

ELEVEN

Life Beyond Sex

This is going to be a short chapter because it pushes against the edges of my current understanding and hopefully offers some food for thought and exploration.

Here's what I currently think is true regarding the potential evolution of sex. First and as discussed previously, our early relationship with sex is a reflection of our conditioning, usually based on desires not unlike those of animals and mostly outside our consciousness. That kind of sex can vary from being lots of fun to incredibly harmful with the primary goal being to get something "I" want, whether power, an orgasm, or a baby. While the sex of youth is most if not all in this category, I venture to say that most humans never move beyond it. Without a way forward, most of us live in that stuck relationship with unsatisfying sex as we enter our mature years, according to my experience and the MRS study.

The beautiful potential of midlife comes when you reframe it, from the end of relevant life as a young fertile woman, to an open field of possibility free from the various limitations of children, work, and stereotypes based in sexism and ageism. From that place, you can explore what I have described previously as the sex of angels based in genuine love, connection, and generosity, with no agenda other than a free expression of love.

Is There Something More?

But here's the "to be continued" part that I learned through my interviews and through speaking with numerous spiritual practitioners and teachers. The sex of angels may still be the "middle way" in the potential evolution of sexuality. Maybe there's even more. Like Vinny said, "It's not the end of the story."

One of the underlying assumptions in this book might seem to be that if you aren't having lots of sex with your partner or yourself, there's something wrong or at least it's a source of suffering that limits the relationship from reaching its full potential. For sure, that's usually the case. Not connecting or not wanting to connect physically with your partner even comes with the medical diagnosis of sexual dysfunction. The term itself implies clearly that there's some level of optimal function that is pathologically lacking. True, not having sex is almost always a symptom of an underlying relationship disconnection. As we've already discussed and the MRS study showed, the degree of dissatisfaction with our sex lives is astonishingly high.

Usually what's lacking is self-awareness, as well as mature love, communication, and connection. One or both members of the partnership are unhappy. They want things to be different. Sometimes someone leaves. Sometimes they gut it out and stay unhappy, and sometimes they seek help. Either way, it's a problem, and the relationship is not being supported and nurtured.

But what if an individual has chosen to be single, or both members of a couple were truly happy and satisfied without having sex frequently or even not at all? What if they don't perceive there to be a problem? Is it possible to have the same degree of intimacy, connection, and expression of love without sex? Is there something beyond sex that is even *more* powerful? And perhaps we need to redefine sex or at least think about whether what's traditionally thought of as sex is too narrow to suit everyone.

Even at my office there is a question on the standard intake form that simply asks "Are you sexually active?" with no further clarification. I'm not quite sure what the point of asking is if we don't get a little more detail, and frankly, does your doctor even want to know? It certainly can feel like the underlying assumption is that the affirmative answer is the healthy choice and the opposite is not. Is it just me, or does that question have a ring of judgment to it?

Caressing For No Reason

Remember my retreats to Ostuni, Italy? It was there that I learned about karezza, which is based on the Italian word for caress. Karezza is a different type of sex that intentionally avoids reaching orgasm. In her book *Cupid's Poison Arrow*, karezza practitioner Marnia Robinson describes that the lack of a goal or end point allows sexual energy to continue to flow indefinitely and may help couples who have become bored with each other to reconnect. When we are always chasing orgasm, performance can become a grind, creating resentment, and disharmony.

The technique of karezza involves cuddling, breathing together with eye contact, and minimal genital stimulation. Obviously it requires a tremendous amount of discipline! This bonding behavior releases the "love hormone" oxytocin but is not associated with the sharp rise (and fall) of dopamine that occurs with orgasm. Dopamine is the same hormone that spikes when we get a hit of our favorite, exciting, addictive passion whether it's a drug, a roller coaster, a bowl of ice cream, or social media. We all know this feels really good temporarily, but the problem is that it always leaves us wishing for more. And with sex, this can lead to a craving for novelty or a feeling of never being really satisfied. In its extreme, this can lead to sex addiction, which like any addiction creates massive harm because the addict puts their needs before the needs of the partner or the relationship. And by definition, addicts are not free.

Some people find karezza by reading about it and just giving it a try. Others have it prescribed to them by a therapist, and some fall across it as an alternative when they can't have sex. Most of the vaginal surgeries I perform, for example, require a six- to eight-week ban on vaginal intercourse, so I encourage couples to improvise. This forced abstinence frequently leads to a great sense of relief and restored connection by being freed from the hamster wheel of monotonous, routine sex. This seems to work particularly well after surgery or illness when circumstances have set up the perfect conditions for caring and compassion. Similarly, when men are experiencing ED, cuddling, massaging, and stroking each other with absolutely no expectation of sex can be remarkably connecting and freeing. For women who would really love a foot or back rub but avoid it since they dread what comes next, what if they knew nothing was going to come next?

Karen described that the relationship dynamics with her husband Matt totally changed after her surgery for pelvic prolapse because he had to take care of her, which was a real role reversal:

> He was really on board with the surgery, and we were both super motivated for it to heal well. So there was no question; we were not having sex until we reached that date on the calendar. After I started feeling better, we missed that closeness. We started just holding each other in bed before we went to sleep, something we truly had never done before. We've been married more than 20 years but cuddling in bed had ever only meant one thing, and that was sex. We even started holding hands again. It was like we were kids falling in love when you're not allowed to go there. That feeling that wells up in your chest when you just really love someone, it's like we had been just jumping right over that and getting down to business.
>
> But when you can't have sex, you can remember what that felt like. I remembered, wow, I really love him. He was taking care of me, and we were just holding each other and thinking, 'Hey, I remember you: the person I fell in love with all those years ago.' In some ways I think just jumping to sex for us felt good, but it bypassed that real heart feeling. Having to slow down and not have an orgasm made us look at that differently. And Matt verbalized, 'I'm not having an orgasm if you're not having one,' so neither of us did. Strange to say, but it was great.

Redefining Sex

Joann and her husband both like to go to spiritual retreats, and while it is usually something they do alone, occasionally they have attended the same one. Particularly at a meditation retreat, sex (including masturbation) is highly discouraged, and men and women are housed separately to make that easier. In the Buddhist tradition, craving is seen as the primary cause of dissatisfaction—the feeling of constantly wanting things to be different than they are and not accepting reality as it is. So, when you are meditating, having an object of desire right next to you can be distracting to say the least.

Knowing and fully accepting that they are not going to have sex that week, there's no point in devoting any energy to thinking about it, and they let it go. In Joann's words:

> It actually feels really freeing. Not needing anything to be different and being completely content with things exactly as they are is perhaps a really good definition of happiness. This is a mutually agreed-upon arrangement, so there is no resentment, and we are each fully supportive of the other in our restraint. Maybe a week or two of abstinence is no big feat, but the point is that it works. In fact, I don't think we ever feel more connected than at a retreat, and our only intimacy takes place by sending each other energy across the room. We don't even need to touch, talk, or make eye contact. There's something about just being completely connected and together, fully present, even with 30 other people in the same room.

The same feeling of heart fullness that Karen described with her husband Matt is able to blossom without some climactic end point. It can last a whole week. Now don't get me wrong, I am not planning to give up sex any time soon, but experimenting with periods of abstinence or non-orgasmic physical connection has been really eye-opening for me. Sex may be one of the best and most available ways for couples to connect genuinely and deeply and express love, but there are other ways. Who knew?

My dad got remarried when he was 78 to an incredible woman several years younger. Penelope was so doting and affectionate, calling him cute names and giving him big hugs and kisses in public. Their relationship was tragically cut short by her death right after Dad's 80th birthday, but their few years together were so sweet, loving, and connected. I just assumed they were sexually active. Actually, Dad later explained, they never had traditional sex and invented their own form of karezza without ever knowing it by that name. Penelope had severe vaginal atrophy and had not been sexually active for more than 20 years, so her vagina was closed for business, and my dad had severe ED that there wasn't much point in treating. Dad explained that they had a beautiful and completely fulfilling sex life nonetheless. They put their bodies together regularly and really connected without ever having penetrative sex. There was absolutely nothing "wrong" that needed to be fixed, and there was no sense of anything missing.

This brings up the issue of redefining what we think of as sex, particularly as more and more people enter their truly elderly years. When a questionnaire asks if you are sexually active, what exactly does that mean? How would Dad and Penelope have answered that question? How would a single person with an active self-pleasuring practice answer that question? Maybe a better question would be, "Are you physically intimate with yourself or a partner?" Sorry Bill Clinton, sex is *definitely* more than vaginal intercourse.

While I don't have the answers to these questions and am just starting to contemplate them myself, what I do know is there's more than one way to skin this cat. The most important thing is consensus if you are in a partnership, and as long as both people are on board and are satisfied, who am I to say what's the "best" way to have sex? Physical intimacy comes in many, many forms. If it is an expression of love, generosity, and connection, everyone is happy. It probably doesn't get any better than that.

> Physical intimacy comes in many, many forms. If it is an expression of love, generosity, and connection, everyone is happy. It probably doesn't get any better than that.

I say "probably" because for most of us, I think that's true. But for a small group of exceptionally evolved humans, I've heard that a uniquely deep spiritual connection can surpass any desire for physical connection. It doesn't mean that sexual desire goes away because we can't escape being sexual beings, but the desire to act on it goes away. In fact, physical connection can become a hindrance to spiritual growth if we believe that any form of wanting or craving prevents peace and freedom. The leaders of many spiritual traditions are expected to adhere to abstinence for that reason, among others.

We all know that abstinence has not worked out so well for religious leaders in many traditions, who instead engaged in sex in covert or illicit ways. But I venture to say that these individuals were not "exceptionally evolved" and have given a bad name to the practice of spiritual abstinence.

Spiritual abstinence only seems to work if it is the culmination of a process of evolution. You cannot jump to it without going through a great deal of personal work and an unusual degree of self-awareness. As with everything, true transformation is a process of traveling a path that is U-shaped. As much as we want to jump from the left to the right of the top of the U, this doesn't result in lasting transformation.

We have to do the work. There is no magic pill, ever.

"And the day came when the risk to remain tight in a bud was more painful than the risk it took to blossom."

—*Anais Nin*

3

THE SECRETS
OF THE
SEXUALLY WOKE

Open to Possibility

Hearing Ben Zander speak about his book *The Art of Possibility* in 2010 totally blew me away. Already in my early-40s, this was the first time I realized that the way I saw the world was severely limited. I credit Zander's talk and book with many things. First, it gave me the impetus to significantly change my career by giving up obstetrics and to overhaul my office culture to help our female providers have some balance and not burn out. It later opened my eyes to exploring various spiritual paths and ultimately to moving on from my first marriage. What if things that I had deemed as impossible actually were possible? What if there was a different way of looking at things that could lead to a better result? As Zander's catchphrase "It's all invented" captures, the way we see the world is almost entirely a product of stories that can—and should—be challenged. This simple tale quoted in his book really opened my eyes.

"A shoe factory sends two marketing scouts to a region of Africa to study the prospects for an expanding business. One sends back a message saying, 'Situation hopeless. No one wears shoes.' The other writes back triumphantly, 'Glorious business opportunity. They have no shoes.'"
—Ben Zander

Life Out of Prison

When it comes to midlife and sexuality, what are the stories that need to be challenged if we want to be among the sexually woke? In as much as these stories are causing harm or are not true, what might be a healthier way to view the same situation?

As an example, let me tell you how this worked for me. In my early-40s, life felt like I was on a conveyor belt going in one direction and largely out of my control. I was driven by a list of things I was supposed to do. Financial planners told me how much money I needed to earn and save to live to 95, to send my kids to an average of six years of private college, and to keep my invented life looking perfect from the outside. We predicted the rise and fall of the stock market for the next 50 years. Every morning, I got up and did what I was supposed to do. I made lots of money, won lots of awards, and made things seem amazing on Facebook.

My then-husband and I had complex wills, life insurance policies, disability policies, and every other imaginable tool to create the illusion that we had this life figured out and under control. I knew the precise date I was going to retire, as well as the date we were going to sell our home. I knew the dates our kids would get married, how much their weddings would cost, when I would become a grandparent, and the date each of us would probably die. Nothing was unknown.

If the goal of all this planning and attempting to manipulate the future was to provide a sense of safety and security, why did the idea of getting old fill me with dread? Why did following this nicely mapped out path feel like I was being buried in an early grave? The fact was I had nothing to look forward to. There was nothing exciting or surprising to anticipate. Life had been wrapped carefully and stuffed into a box. Looking into the future felt like looking down a long, dark, narrowing tunnel. It was a death march.

At that same time, I was struggling with getting older. I was getting crow's feet. Gray hairs became too many to pluck out. My sex drive was non-existent. Women much younger than me were enjoying leadership roles and accolades and were prominently featured in the media. I could feel myself slowly being pushed out of the picture of what matters.

After hearing Ben Zander talk, the wall of that tunnel started to be a little more opaque. A little light started to come in. If there was light on the other side of those tunnel walls, what was out there? I read Zander's book, and my curiosity started to rise. Within a few months, I was devouring a book every week and attending every seminar I could find on the subject of personal growth and spirituality. As my self-invented tunnel started to crumble, the future began to look quite different: an open field of possibility, openness, emptiness—a blank canvas ready for me to paint.

The degree to which this changed my life cannot be overstated, and all I did was change my perspective. Nothing "out there" changed. The only thing that changed was my ability to see it. I woke up.

Here's an observation from 20 years as a gynecologist and 52 years as a woman. When you feel trapped in a box, you don't want to have sex. Truly making love is generative, free, expressive, and creative. It's a dance that takes place in an open field, not a dark tunnel. Love cannot be confined within walls. Trying to do so makes it die.

This observation points to one of the key findings of my research and perhaps the most important "secret." It's not aging that causes our sex lives to decline. It's the feeling, conscious or subconscious, that we are trapped.

This is why women of all ages invariably have a spike in libido when they start a new relationship and why having a deep spiritual understanding (of something bigger than ourselves) is associated with a better sex life. The truth is we are not and never were trapped. We put ourselves in a prison but forget we hold the key. Outside those walls is a world of infinite possibility.

Sex in the New World

As I talked with the sexually woke, this theme came up over and over again. These women did not complain about aging, rather they appreciated their newfound wisdom and freedom and universally described this as the best time of their lives. Surprisingly to me, many women shared similar images and metaphors to describe their own awakening. In Robin's words:

 The idea of the fullness in life when we are younger is paradoxical because we tend to think of fullness related to success, achievement, money, and status. Then we find the futility when we get to menopause—the futility of trying to hold it all together. The first half of my life, I felt like I was building a very solid structure. That gave me some comfort. But then we literally start to see our bodies fall apart and realize that it's all falling apart really. That solid structure was not based in anything real. My new house got old, my perfect kids grew up and didn't do what the plan dictated, and my marriage fell apart. For me, the acceptance of that and letting go of the fantasy of solidity really let me enter the fullness of life. With the solidity of the walls I had created, I had no access to other possibilities. I was pretty delusional that life was solid.

After my divorce, I was free—finally free to have that fullness of life and be available to meet someone I could be my full self with as my full sexual being. I'm 55, and life has never been better. As for sex, I'm only just beginning to find out where I can go with that. There's no road map, no walls. I can go wherever I want. It's beautiful.

All of a sudden you have some space. You can finally ask those questions like, "What am I really here to do?" With that space to reflect, you can integrate yourself, pull all those pieces together, and really show up. People might call it a midlife crisis, saying, "Oh, she went nuts, left her husband, and moved to France." But I don't think that's what it is. It's an awakening. More like: "Oh, I've only been half here all this time." When you've cut off your sexual being and then find it, it's like you've been walking around without one arm then realizing that you have both. "Wow! Look at all these things I can do now with two arms!"

Alexa shares another beautiful metaphor:

I think of my sexuality as a sea snail, the kind with the coiled shell. For most of my life, my sexuality had lived inside a shell. For one thing, it's not safe to be gay, so I hid. But now when I feel safe and happy, the snail will venture out of her shell and start to venture across the ocean floor and explore this unknown new world. I used to think the shell was a prison, but it's really just a place to be safe if there's real harm around. When I feel safe, there's a door that I can venture out of and go as far as I want.

I'm 61, and I was thinking about women my age whose sexuality has gone out like the tide or at least they think it has. Then I started thinking about spaciousness, to live in the spaciousness of the unknown, of possibility. Inside the shell can feel safer, but I think an existence with spaciousness is what we are hopefully evolving into. There's this 'letting go of certainty' aspect in sexuality that mirrors letting go into the spiritual life. For me, I think that's how those two come together. There's a huge element of letting go around the time of menopause. The reality of our finite life can be very freeing. There's a letting go of needing to be a certain way, the way that conforms to being young. Instead of framing that as loss, to me it's letting go of a whole lot of baggage and realizing your shell has a door. It's freedom. 99

I was amazed at how frequently words like "freedom" and "liberation" were used by the sexually woke in relation to midlife. This certainly wasn't what I was taught! Freedom came in many forms: freedom from limiting beliefs, freedom from fear of pregnancy, and even freedom to make more noise or be more spontaneous without family in the house. Christine adds:

Sex is so liberating now. I am past the baby stage. There's no more waiting for a period to either get here or not and no more worrying about getting pregnant. I know what I like, and we are comfortable with each other. His body knows my body; it 'listens,' and it's learned when to move left or right, keep going, stop, or try something else. Although we talk openly about sex, sometimes he just knows exactly what to do by the way my body is responding. It's like we are in our 20s again but better because we've both learned so much and look forward to just being together. 99

As Caitlin describes:

It seems to me there are two possibilities. One is that you are still in a fog of years of youthful, idiotic, and delusional thinking, not really understanding things. On the other hand, now with some years and experience under your belt, you have a certain strength, clarity, and wisdom. I am starting to understand things. In the old days, they would have called me a crone. The wise old woman that the village would go to for advice. But maybe I can be a sexy crone. I feel better than ever. I don't care so much what other people think. I am free to be myself. I can make love with my husband, and I am all here. "

Another kind of freedom was described in several ways by the sexually woke: freedom from the male "gaze." This was one type of freedom that had not occurred to me previously. I work in an almost entirely female world. My patients and co-workers are women and rarely does discomfort with issues like sexual harassment and personal safety come up in my professional world. But for many women, this has been a constant reality that thankfully fades with age. Maryann puts it this way:

" I just think midlife comes with a sort of ease, a comfort in your own being. I still have some body image issues but way less than when I was young. It's the ease with which we wear our lives. I can 'wear my life as a loose garment.' I like that saying. It's not giving up; it's letting go. I no longer have to look good for men, I'm not getting catcalls when I walk down the street, and I'm not getting hit on at work. I'm not getting harassed. There's so much freedom in that. I'm not a slave to my period or to anyone else. I don't have to live up to some ridiculous standard that has us measure ourselves through the eyes of men. Now I can measure myself with my own stick. I look good for myself. "

No Time to Rush

I previously mentioned Tara Brach, one of my favorite authors, speakers, and teachers. A long-time psychotherapist, she shared a story from one of her clients who had been diagnosed with cancer and told that her life would be cut short. Suddenly realizing the importance of every day, she told Tara that instead of rushing to get things done in her limited time, she slowed down to savor each moment. "I have no time to rush," she said. While Tara didn't share about this woman's sex life, one can imagine that it grew richer and more fulfilling as did every aspect of life.

One common realization in midlife is that we are all going to die. Even you. Even me. A common cultural response to this realization is to try to deny it, backpedaling furiously to try to be younger, fueled by the fear that *I don't have enough time.* But for the sexually woke, the universal response was something different. Back to the idea of love and fear, they approached their limited time with a sense of love, openness, and ease. In Kimberly's words:

> I think there are two choices when we go through menopause. There's 'Oh God. I'm going to die soon' with a negative, fearful view of the future. Like 'I'm old now, so I may as well give up.' That's pretty bleak. But the other way is 'Oh gosh. We don't have forever. Let's make the most out of every moment.' Every day is more precious. It opens you up to see the things that have been there all the time and let go of the stuff that makes you miserable. One day, one of us will not be here. I don't worry about the little things anymore. I let them go. Life is too short to bicker. We don't want to have regrets that we didn't take the opportunity to enjoy each other and give to each other. I think that's what we realized as we got older. I wouldn't trade this time in my life for anything at all.

Live from Abundance

All of these accounts seem to point to one thing: a shift from a scarcity mentality based in fear, to an abundance mentality based in love and freedom. Whatever metaphor was used—emerging from a box or a tunnel, coming out of a shell, finding freedom and spaciousness, becoming more present in the moment, having more peace and ease—the sexually woke did not see themselves as old and irrelevant. They did not view their lives as being over; rather they had a strong sense of a new beginning. Reverend Linda sums this up so well:

> I remember having joyful, completely free sex when we were trying to have a baby. It was a very liberating time. You're kind of going to that creative place. But I think post-menopausal sex is also about liberation. It's not about procreation anymore, but it's expressive of other things, other longings. A word we use in the marriage rite is 'cherish.' In this season, I am really coming to cherish my husband. I'm almost 60, and I've been so aware that he's not going to be around forever. The sense of preciousness around that is really interesting to me. From a theological perspective, sex is generative but not just in the

way of procreation. It should give you life and give life to others through your love for each other.

In our tradition, we talk about the 'three goods' of marriage, which are also in the marriage vows. Marriage is for the mutual joy of the couple, for help and comfort in adversity and prosperity, and for procreation. So the first two remain as we age. Mutual joy, help and comfort, no matter what. Sex can be an expression of mutual joy. That feels very liberating. The way my husband adores me, I have never been adored by anyone like that. His adoration, his love, has made so much of my life possible. So it's creative, it's generative, way after having babies is the goal. I think many people in the spiritual world see sex as an encumbrance rather than a resource. I think that's a misunderstanding.

Thanks, Linda. I think so too.

Know Yourself First

We already talked about the cliché that you have to love yourself before you can love anyone else, at least in the way the sexually woke showed me how to love. What came up in some form in every interview was a deep understanding of the importance of approaching relationships from a position of wholeness. Without it, genuine, lasting connection and intimacy just don't seem to be possible. The shift from codependence to co-creation seems to be absolutely vital if we want to have a vibrant love life that doesn't die of old age.

Finding out who you are and getting to know yourself is the adventure of a lifetime and was unpacked earlier in the book. It's one of those things that you can't believe you lived without once you find it. The words of "Amazing Grace" come to mind. "I once was lost but now am found, was blind but now I see." Whatever your religious background, this is a powerful message about waking up to who you are and seeing what was there all along: a beautiful, perfect human being.

The Catch-22

I personally tried for most of my life to define myself through the eyes of others. Through my own experience and my research, I can tell you this never ends well. Until you can define yourself through your own eyes and love yourself exactly as you are, it's impossible for you to accept that from someone else. Just do the math. If I'm unlovable, then I'm unlovable. There's no way to fix unlovability by having someone else love you. They can't truly love you because you are unlovable. It's a catch-22. I think Denise puts it perfectly:

> The sex is sort of a symptom of how well the relationship is doing. If you have all the parts in place, and you've done the work on yourself, then—and only then—are you going to be free to have a healthy sexual relationship. I think some people—most people—go about it the wrong way. They're trying to have a healthy sexual relationship, but they haven't done the work on themselves that's going to allow that to be possible. It's like we are always trying to take a shortcut, but there's no shortcut. If you don't really understand what makes you tick and if you don't have control over your reactions, then you really can't be in a healthy relationship. We look to relationships to fix these things for us. Someone else can't do that for you. They have their own self to manage. You have to do your own work. Period.

I heard this message from so many people in so many different ways. If you are coming into a relationship full of self-hatred or self-doubt and you are not completely integrated or pulled together, you really can't show up as a full participant in a relationship. You don't know yourself yet. So how can you expect anyone else to? In Veronica's experience:

> When you don't have yourself figured out, that is so selfish. You don't have anything to give. You are pulling from the other person for every need you have in your life. It's a terrible burden to put on the relationship, to be needy like that. You are like another child, another mouth to feed, instead of a partner who brings something valuable to the table. It's going to be a strain on top of a strain. I've been there. It was terrible. I had to get independent and figure myself out. Or it will chase them off or cause a mess of conflict for sure.

Filling Our Own Hole

Whatever damage was done to you by your caretakers, partners, teachers, coworkers, church, or whomever, at some point it's time to stop complaining and just take control back. It feels good for a while to sit in a corner and complain about all the harm that was done to you. Believe me, I spent more than 30 years in that place, and I understand. My poor parenting and list of injustices gave me every right to complain. But the problem was, it didn't help. Solidifying myself in the victim role gave me no solace other than the temporary relief of feeling self-righteous. But there's no lasting happiness in being a victim.

Using the model that I love so much from the Conscious Leadership Group, we need to shift from the place of *to me* to the place of *by me* to find peace and contentment. We need to take back control of our lives by assuming full responsibility for where we are. Not many people are brave enough to do that which is why the sexually woke was a mere 7 percent. But there is hope. Take a breath. If someone can do it, then you can do it. The sexually woke do not share any magic superpowers. They are not especially thin, tall, or rich. They are just like you. They are regular people who, for whatever reason, decided to listen to and act on that whisper from within that was telling them there was more to life.

How do you get yourself out of decades of habits and conditioning? How do you start to let go of the story of yourself and everyone else? How do you move toward changes that will lead you to this world of possibility? Perhaps listening to the wise words of the sexually woke will help guide you.

Christine remembers:

> I used to say to myself, 'I hate you. You are so stupid!' when I did something wrong or hurt someone's feelings. I had to reprogram myself. There's a song, 'The Noise in Your Head'—you have to play a different song—'I love you. I love you.' Once I started playing a different song, I had to stop saying those words and even stop thinking them. Instead of 'You are so stupid,' I played a new song. I made a mistake, but I am a good person and love myself unconditionally. I am forgiven. If I tell myself something positive like that, which is the truth, loving and positive people will gravitate towards me. I'll have more positive people in my life. I realized I was responsible for that mess. Maybe I didn't start it, but I kept it going by believing it. And only I can get myself out of it.
>
> As women we are taught to give, give, give. But I can't save anyone else if we're both drowning. Sometimes you have to set boundaries and put yourself first. If that's selfish, then I guess I am selfish. But if I am going to give to others, I have to take care of myself first. I have to love myself first.

Helen describes her new happiness like this:

> I'm not looking for my husband to fulfill me. I'm not looking for anything in the world to make me happy because I know that's not possible. I know that I am perfect and whole in myself. All happiness is within me. Consequently, I don't have unrealistic expectations that can't be met by anything or anyone. If I'm not happy, it's something in me. It's not because he said or did something. That's a very peaceful life when two people feel the same way. We have that understanding because we're not looking to someone else to make something happen. There's this cycle people get in of expectation and disappointment when they don't live up to our fantasy for how they are 'supposed' to be. I don't expect him to be perfect; he doesn't expect me to be perfect. It's okay. We are human. We just forgive and move on to another day.

Jackie puts it this way:

> One of my big insights is that no one can fill the hole. You have to fill it from the inside out; then a relationship with another person is just an icing on the cake kind of thing. When you're in a position to fill that hole for yourself, you can be easy with the other person. The clinging is not there so much. You can let that person be free, and you can be free. You can be much more accepting of them because you don't really need them. They are just an added something to your life.
>
> After I got divorced, I felt like I was always considered a second-class citizen being single, especially being single and older. I'm 65. I can see people sometimes have this look of pity for me. It's like, 'Oh, poor thing. Do we need to help you find somebody?' I mean, it is really a precarious situation to need someone to make you happy. What happens when they are gone? You're kind of doomed. It's really about loneliness. I enjoy being alone sometimes, but I don't call it loneliness. I call it solitude, peace. I'm not ruling out another relationship, but I don't need it. I like my own company. I think that makes me much more attractive actually, at least to anyone who I would want to be with.

The Math of Withholding

Here's some simple logic. You can't really be with someone if you aren't fully present. I guess that goes without saying. You also can't be fully present if you're harboring unspoken feelings or hiding the truth because you're not showing yourself. In as much as you are withholding something of yourself—maybe you're stuck in resentment or trying to be straight or skinny or light skinned or (fill in the blank)—that situation makes it impossible for someone to know you. If you're not expressing your full true self, then how can you be in a genuine, connected relationship? If you're half a person presenting to another half a person, you're going to bump up against each other like bumper cars. There will be no real connection. That describes most of my first marriage right there. Alexa adds beautifully:

> If there's an elephant in the room—you know, this thing you would be fighting about if you dared to fight—but you just pretend to ignore it, then the elephant is stepping all over the potted plants. While you are ignoring the elephant, it's killing everything. That's the kind of thing that makes it impossible for me to relax into love and sexuality, just the lack of being real and seeing what's in the room and dealing with it. Elephants are not evil, but they need to be dealt with, or they will destroy your house.

Alexa is so right about that. Maybe five or 10 years before I got divorced, my then-husband would want to talk about sex, but I couldn't talk about it. I would say, "Just leave it alone. It will get better when the kids are older. This is normal. Trust me; I'm a gynecologist. Talking about it just makes it worse." I knew there was something about our relationship that would fall apart if we talked about it, and I wasn't ready for that. Talk about an elephant in the room.

Taking the Reins

In the end, you're responsible for your own pleasure, sexual and otherwise. No one else is going to create that for you. Here's a possibly useful metaphor. I happen to love exercise, and while I know that's not common, I often compare sex to exercise when I think about things that take work but have incredible benefits. To get the benefit of exercise, you have to exercise; you have to do the work. Think about golf or tennis. You can't just study it, read about it, or look at pictures, and before you do it with someone else, it's useful to practice it by yourself. Along those lines, Denise describes:

> When I go to yoga, it's like you step out of your life and have such good fortune to be able to walk into a room and focus on you, which is such bliss for someone who has been taking care of kids, jobs, and whatnot. It's such a luxury. What if we could just convince ourselves that sex can be the same? If we could be more aware, it's not just a male feeling that we respond to, but it's a female feeling as well. We can cultivate it just like we cultivate yoga or exercise and get better at cultivating that feeling. I think the more we cultivate it by ourselves, the more we will know ourselves, so we can attend to our sexual needs and be more present for our husbands or partners.

When I asked Christine what advice she would give to other women, she offers:

> I would say, without a doubt, you have to learn how to give yourself an orgasm. Once you can give yourself an orgasm, you might realize, what do I need you for? I might like you or love you, but I don't need you. Learn to make yourself happy. There's something about a woman who can walk around and say, 'Hey, I'm happy.' Then you'll attract the right man. The thing is happiness doesn't come from some external source. You have to win it yourself, otherwise you will become a hostage . . . a hostage to a bad marriage or a hostage to the idea that it's bad to be alone. I'd rather be alone than to be mistreated by someone. I love my husband, and I can't imagine that he would do anything to blindside me, but if he does, I know how to walk away.

We already talked about vibrators and toys in Part 1 of this book. I can tell you almost without exception, the sexually woke knew how to take pleasure into their own hands. After being on the low end of the power differential since the beginning of time, taking control of your sexual pleasure can be enormously empowering.

Jill has a spot-on perspective:

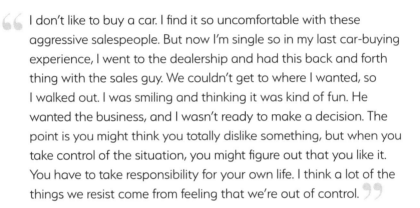

> I don't like to buy a car. I find it so uncomfortable with these aggressive salespeople. But now I'm single so in my last car-buying experience, I went to the dealership and had this back and forth thing with the sales guy. We couldn't get to where I wanted, so I walked out. I was smiling and thinking it was kind of fun. He wanted the business, and I wasn't ready to make a decision. The point is you might think you totally dislike something, but when you take control of the situation, you might figure out that you like it. You have to take responsibility for your own life. I think a lot of the things we resist come from feeling that we're out of control.

Perhaps this comes down to one thing. You are not a victim, and life is not happening to you. Whatever it is, it's not personal. Victims are not free. Those at the mercy of the world are not free. Once you truly know yourself and can take 100 percent responsibility for where you are in life, you are free. Free to love and be loved, exactly as you are.

Intention and Attention

Zen Master Richard Baker Roshi was once asked to summarize how to guide humans toward true transformation. His answer was very simple. "Transformation is caused by two things—Intention and Attention." Said another way, "The grass is always greener where you water it."

So what's the difference between intention and attention anyway? To me, intention comes from a deep internal decision to act in a certain way on purpose. Attention, on the other hand, describes where I choose to focus my mind. Similar but different.

Coming and Going

As I spoke to the sexually woke, one thing became very clear. Their relationships had not grown stronger and closer by accident. They were not particularly blessed or lucky, and none had escaped considerable suffering and struggle. Many had been through painful divorces and were in a second or third marriage. And all had suffered painful and difficult times in their current relationships. What they shared in common was a deep intention to place value on the current relationship, to make the relationship a priority, and to pay attention both to each other and to the relationship as a separate organism.

One of my favorite questions, which developed as the interviews progressed, was how the couple marked coming and going. In other words, I was interested if they had a ritual around saying goodbye and hello, goodnight and good morning. Without exception, every woman in the sexually woke group described a ritual that included an intentional pause in activity to become present and to say hello and goodbye with an expression of love. Every. Single. Time. This small daily moment of presence, attention, and recognition seemed to keep the fire of love alive.

There's something magical about being with another human and knowing you have that person's full attention, even if for a minute. That daily expression of importance and acknowledgment of "we're good" is both priceless and so easy to deliver. This might be the single easiest thing that you might commit to if you want to become more connected. The only requirement is being vulnerable 30 seconds each day. There's so much to gain, and what do you have to lose?

Jill and Adam always make a point of having a kiss goodnight and an "I love you" before they go to sleep, allowing him to roll over on his left side (he has an old injury to his right shoulder) and away from her without her feeling abandoned. Similarly, neither of them leaves the house without a hug and a kiss, and they drop what they are doing to greet the other upon arrival home.

Jill says:

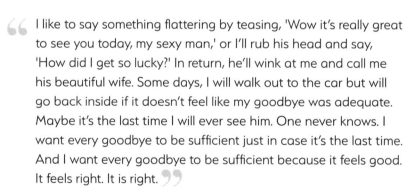

> I like to say something flattering by teasing, 'Wow it's really great to see you today, my sexy man,' or I'll rub his head and say, 'How did I get so lucky?' In return, he'll wink at me and call me his beautiful wife. Some days, I will walk out to the car but will go back inside if it doesn't feel like my goodbye was adequate. Maybe it's the last time I will ever see him. One never knows. I want every goodbye to be sufficient just in case it's the last time. And I want every goodbye to be sufficient because it feels good. It feels right. It is right.

This was really a common theme. The sexually woke were genuinely happy to see each other and made a point to vocalize that emotion. I didn't hear descriptions of sadness or fear when the other left since the sexually woke did not cling to or feel needy around their partners. They had moved from codependence to co-creation. There was recognition of value, a genuine shift of focus to the other, and a wish for the other to have happiness in whatever they were doing that day.

Elizabeth shares a sweet daily routine. After almost 30 years of marriage, she said every day starts out the same:

> We have a morning ritual. It's not that we decided it was a ritual, but it just happened. Pretty much every morning when we wake up, he rolls over, pulls me to him, and holds me just for a minute, maybe while the alarm is snoozing. He says, 'You are such a beautiful wife. I love you.' Whatever happened yesterday doesn't matter. This is a new day. Pretty much every day, this man has done that. It's just a little thing, but we start our day knowing 'I am important to you, this is going to be a good day, and we are good.' I think most people just jump out of bed and get out the door. The alarm goes off, and their mind is already at the office. I mean, what's the point of working so hard if you end up getting divorced? There's no recognition that we are important, you are important.

When Jill says goodbye to Adam, "Have a good day, darling" isn't a trite remark coming from her thinking brain; it's a genuine wish coming from her heart:

> To get to that place, I have to pause for a second, become present, find my body, and speak from the heart. It takes intention. I do it because it's important. He is important to me. Words as simple as 'hello' and 'goodbye' can be said from many places and can mean many things. My intention is to say them from the heart and with presence as a whole-body statement.
>
> Contrast this with my first marriage in which the first things out of my mouth when I got home were, 'Hey, did you take the trash out? Is the nanny still here? Did you pay that credit card bill?' Usually he would walk right past me and go upstairs. If I had been naked doing a pole dance, he wouldn't have noticed. There was zero recognition by either side of another fragile, beautiful human that needed acknowledgment, attention, and love.

This is how relationships die. Many MRS participants had similar stories. Alison laughs:

> When Darren comes home, our two dogs get really excited. After 20 years together, he'll be like, 'Hey guys, get out of my way because I can't get to mom and give her a kiss!'

Christina describes:

> Whenever my husband walks in, I tell him, 'Hey, it's good to see you! You're home from work!' and I give him a hug. I want him to feel like he's home, this is his safe place where he is loved, and that he's worthy to be hugged and kissed and touched.

Valuing Connection

The sexually woke also share deep intention to have regular sexual connection or even a non-sexual intimate connection. It might be a long hug, a passionate kiss, or a deep look into each other's eyes. The priority to be intimate comes before almost everything else. When many of us put it off until later, the sexually woke put intimacy at or near the top of the list. More than sex, they prioritized quality time together and put intention into being connected.

Carla describes that after having a baby in her early-40s, she was still determined to keep the fire burning with Michael:

> I had to put intentional effort into making sure it was still part of our lives. That's the key. I would tell him, 'Let's still be intimate together, but we will just have to get creative because right now, I don't want to be touched. My breasts hurt, and my vagina is dry. But I still want to be connected. I still want to be intimate. I still want to be sexual but maybe not as often. If you still want to be sexual, I get it. I want to participate in some form or fashion. Let's just do a hand job, and I'll kiss you because I don't want to be touched down there. I still love watching you have an orgasm. Maybe I don't want one right now, so let's not go there, or maybe if I do feel like one, we might have to do something different, and I'll show you what works.'

Rosie and her husband travel a lot for work and have to make the most of their time together:

> When I'm back in town, we need time for us to spend together, and we laugh because sex is our shortcut. We can sit down and have an intellectual conversation and a meal, or we can have sex. Sometimes we will have sex at night or sometimes in the morning. It's a priority, and we know we don't have much time. Then it's like, 'Oh, I've got to get on a plane,' so the night before we'd have sex, and in the morning we'd have sex. We have to get it in since we're not going to have it again for a couple of weeks. It's like our accelerator for connection. We could sit down and have a glass of wine and talk all night, but if we just make love first, we are connecting, and we can just go from there.

Fifty-nine-year-old Karen has been married for 40 years. She describes:

> If you let it happen by accident, it's not going to happen. You have to make it intentional. If you wait until you go to bed, everyone is tired. You need to acknowledge, 'Whatever I need to do, that little extra laundry, it can wait. Let's go to bed a little earlier tonight if we can. I can do laundry after if it's that important.' I need to make sure I'm not so exhausted—and same for him—that we get to bed and admit, 'Well, we were going to have sex, but we're just too tired.'
>
> We want to say to the other person, 'I am making time for you because you are very important.' It's not necessarily the act of sex. It's that I am sharing myself with you even at my most vulnerable point at the end of a busy day because I value you that much. I think this is important for us. Plus it's fun. It makes us lighten up and have a giggle. Otherwise we are telling our partner, 'You're not as important as the laundry. You're not as important as the children. I'll get to you after all those things. Right now, I'm too tired.' How does that feel? Not very good. Life gets so serious. Then we wonder why marriages don't work or why people look elsewhere for intimacy.

> I remember my husband reading an article in the paper that said, 'Your kids are not the most important thing. Your partner was here before them, and the two of you are the foundation for the family. You need to value your relationship first.' I'm like, 'You're right about that.'
>
> The thing I would like to tell people is when you are together, just be together. Even if you are watching TV together, watch TV together. Don't be on the phone or having another conversation.

That's incredibly important advice. When you are together, be present. Turn off your phone. If your mind is somewhere else, then you are not giving yourself to that person. It's like being half there. We all know that feeling when someone isn't really there. It tells us, "You are not that important":

> When someone is really, really present with you, it's a gift. They are choosing you above all the other billion things in the world. You feel important and loved. You are important and loved.

Prioritizing Your Relationship

It's taken my whole life to believe Karen and her husband are wise to prioritize their relationship, not the kids. It's counter-cultural to say so, but without a strong, connected parental or adult relationship as the central focus, the kids will suffer. We are not doing our kids any favors by putting ourselves last and focusing on their every whim. We are raising a generation of kids who see adults not valuing themselves and their partners, and they will model that behavior. Kids learn much more from watching what we do than from hearing what we say. We are sending mixed messages to them: they should value themselves, but we don't value ourselves.

I want to teach my kids and later my grandkids that I am valuable, and I value myself. This will empower them to cultivate their own sense of worth and belonging from within rather than needing it from outside sources in the form of excessive praise or being spoiled. If they see me taking time for myself, treating myself with care and attention, and treating my relationship with care and attention, my hope is they will carry this into adulthood and become strong, resilient, and self-compassionate individuals prepared to enter into healthy, long-term relationships.

The sexually woke share a deep recognition that genuine caring for their partner's well-being as well as sex and intimacy are vital for the relationship. There is a deep desire for their partner to be fulfilled and a deep wanting to be fulfilled as well. This takes time and effort that is directly proportional to the value placed on the relationship. I recall in my first marriage, I put all of my energy into work, the kids, and training for triathlons. At one point, my then-husband said, "If you put half of the energy into me that you put into your work and hobbies, things would be great between us." He may have been right. This is a perfect example of effort mirroring the value placed on the relationship. I didn't value the relationship, and I didn't take care of it. I took it for granted.

We take care of the things we value. We give them time, effort, and presence. Alison notes:

> We talk about this. Sex is very important to my husband. We have been married for 20 years, but he still feels sex is an expression of the fact that I love him, I care about him, and I want to be with him. I can cook him dinner, I can clean the house, and I can do his laundry, but for him, his love language is sex. We are going to live until say 85 or 90. That's a long time if you give up at 50. I know some women do that. I think part of giving up is because society says, 'You're at that age now. You're in menopause, and that's just the way things are.' It takes energy to move forward and beyond that. If your hormones are out of whack and you don't feel good, you've got to do something. My marriage is important.

Similarly, Victoria describes:

> After the kids are gone, it's just going to be you and your husband. You put everything else on the calendar, so why not put yourselves on the calendar? If you love your marriage enough, you need to put it on the calendar at least every week. Every day, really. I feel like it's important to spend quality time together every day, even if it's not sex. It's just like the garden. If you don't tend to that garden, it's going to get full of weeds and die. Sex should connect you.
>
> It's a connecting tool. I notice that if I don't get enough or he doesn't get enough, we get a little grouchy. It's like, 'Okay, it's time.'

When Joann doesn't have sex for a week or two, she says that something feels off:

> No matter what else is going on, intentionally making sure we get in a quickie if it's really busy always resets our connection. Sometimes we will both be getting ready for work, and I'll just take off my clothes and say, 'Let's do it. We might not have time tonight. I can be five minutes late!' Or if I'm downstairs getting breakfast, he will text me and say, 'Want to come upstairs for a few minutes?' When one of us is away on a trip, we might have phone sex, text sex, or a fantasy chat. I want to have that, and I want him to have it. Even when we are on opposite sides of the world, we can still come together in deep connection. And sex is not always intercourse or orgasm. Sometimes a long hug, a pat on the bottom, or a cuddle on the couch will suffice, but without that regular physical connection, things get out of balance.

The Role of Self-Care

The sexually woke ubiquitously pay attention to advocating for themselves. Sometimes that means intentionally carving out time for self-care. Valuing self-care pretty much abolishes codependent behaviors, which stem from the unconscious desire to be a hero or martyr. Constantly catering to the other person's needs to the detriment of both parties sets the stage for codependence. Conversely, making self-care and time alone intentional seems to dramatically improve sexual connection. This might seem counter-intuitive, but it's one of the most important lessons I have ever learned. As Christina points out:

> Intentional self-care means you are worth it. I can go to a movie by myself or go for a walk and just clear my mind. Then I am ready to give myself fully to my family when I get home, to be present and really listen to them and be with them. For my birthday, my husband asked me what I wanted, and I said, 'I want to go to Hawaii without you and the kids.' I don't think there's anything wrong with that, but we are taught we need to be together every moment. I just don't think that's healthy. I like me. I need to spend some time with me. Sometimes I set a goal for myself, like

trying to run a mile in eight minutes. Or *yo estudio espanol con Rosetta Stone*. Whatever floats your boat. To learn something new, when I am excited about that, it filters into everything. Then I'm excited about seeing my kids coming through the door, and I've got something exciting to share with my husband. If you find something that makes you happy, it will filter into your relationships and into the bedroom.

Vanessa shares:

My husband says I'm beautiful, but I'd like to lose 20 pounds for myself. I exercise. I eat right. When I do the stuff I like to do and stay active, I feel better mentally, and my body responds to that sexually. I think it's important to feel good about yourself no matter what size you are. I got breast implants when I was 53. It's like I can't get my stomach smaller, so I'm going to get proportional. If it makes you feel better about yourself, it makes you feel more desirable and makes you feel more like having sex. It's kind of a snowball effect.

For me, self-care means continuing to focus on what I'm personally passionate about and my own path of self-discovery separate from a partner. I might go to a meditation retreat, take the dogs to the beach for a long walk, or commit to a triathlon—for myself. These things make me feel whole and that I'm worth investing time in.

Joann says it this way:

I go on trips by myself or with girlfriends. He does the same thing, perhaps traveling to Thailand or Peru by himself for a personal adventure, riding his motorcycle (which the old me said he could never have, but who am I to restrict what makes him happy, and what does that say about me?), or just working out at the gym, which he loves to do alone. Both of us have friends that are not shared as well as mutual ones, and that's okay.

When we can pay attention to our own needs and come together as two whole, satisfied people who are committed to supporting each other's development, our sex life is on fire. We can't give what we don't have. When we feel depleted or unable to find a moment for ourselves, it takes a real willingness and intention to step outside that paradigm and proclaim, 'I am worth it.' 🙶

One thing that came up frequently in my interviews was the importance of having friendships outside the primary relationship, especially same-sex friends. Many of us lose touch with friends when kids are occupying all of our time, but midlife can offer a wonderful opportunity to reconnect with old friends or cultivate new ones. My very first girls' trip was recently to Europe for a friend's 50th birthday. I made time for it and prioritized it, and boy was it worth it! Depending on one person for close connection is precarious and can create a feeling of weight or being trapped. As Veronica puts it:

> I struggled a bit finding a good friend once everyone got so busy with their own lives. Your spouse may be your best friend, but they cannot be the only one. It's so important to have a meaningful life apart from your spouse as well. It's so good if you can find a woman friend whom you can really trust. She's like gold. I have about five friends now, and I feel very blessed. If you have one, you are blessed, but I had one, and she introduced me to the next one. That's really important. Someone else to talk to who is not your spouse and not your kids. People can add so much to your life if you invite them in. When my husband and I are both happy and not depending on each other for everything, things work so much better in our relationship. 🙶

When I feel good about myself and follow my own path with authenticity, only then can I show up as a fully engaged and present partner. It has to be a priority. There have been times in my own relationships when this has slipped, and I have seen the negative repercussions.

Jill describes it this way:

> At times, both of us have felt that we're losing our individual selves into the relationship when we didn't focus enough attention on our own needs and didn't support the other's focus on fulfilling their needs. In one particularly rough patch, I was told in no uncertain terms, 'You know, this is not the Jill Show. I feel like one

giant support blanket. I want to feel loved and supported too. I'm living your life. I want my life back!' Ouch! Feedback received. I wanted his life back, too, and we set our intentions to undo the circumstances that had caused him to feel that way. I refocused my attention on being present for him in a way that supported his growth rather than smothering it.

Small Acts with Big Impact

Small acts of kindness are inevitably valued highly by the sexually woke, and the impact of these small acts carries a big bang. Alexa says:

> The one thing I totally love is he'll take my car and drive me to work. He'll pick me up at night. If it's rainy or cold or whatever it is, I know my car with him driving it is right out there, and I don't have to walk all the way across the parking lot in the cold, in the dark, or the wet. That's just so sweet. The small moments of caring add up in an amazing way. It's not the great, dramatic instances that punctuate an otherwise self-centered life. It's lots of these small things that make it work.

Similarly, Alison describes:

> The little things you do that you might think are insignificant are probably really significant. I'll look at my husband and say, 'You are just so cute.' He'll smile and say, 'I'm glad you think so. Okay, do you want to have sex? Is that it?' We have a lot of fun with words. I think if you don't feel like doing that, maybe it's not the right person.

Paying attention to what makes your partner happy might seem like a little thing, but it means a lot to the sexually woke. Elizabeth suggests:

> Find out the top five things each person wants, and if you both take care of those five things, then you're good to go. I know what makes my husband happy. He loves espresso. So I make sure we have a good assortment of espresso and make time to enjoy it. He really likes great-quality bacon on the weekends. So every Friday, I go out and make sure we have some. He does the same for the

things I love. It makes me want to make love to him. That also keeps him happy.

To keep your man happy might be stupid things. I think most women know what they are, but they don't care. They are like, 'I don't give a shit.' I don't know what holds people back from that kind of generosity; maybe it's just selfishness or like, 'I'm not going to do that for you because you don't do that for me.' Then nobody goes first, and everyone is stuck. Just go first, for God's sake. 99

Carla is 46 and has been married to her second husband for eight years and is still deeply in love:

66 He buys me flowers for no reason at the grocery store, possibly just because the ones he bought me last week died. 99

Maria is 63, and her husband still leaves her sticky love notes on the bathroom mirror:

66 Sometimes he will make the little sticky notes into a heart. He just makes me feel so appreciated. 99

Aww. Maria adds:

66 When we are at our best, he notices when I am feeling stressed or time pressured and will say something like, 'What can I do for you today, darling? Why don't I pick up the kids from school so you can get your workout in?' Or he will hand-wash my car as a surprise and not tell me or buy me some pickled beets (my favorite). I'll write lipstick notes on the mirror when he's been gone for a few days. These are small things that take no time or effort. What they do take is intention, and they are priceless. Personally, I would rather have a surprise car wash than diamond jewelry. Anyone can buy a diamond. Not many men will do a surprise car wash. That's a labor of love that stems from the heart. 99

Novelty as a Firestarter

Intentionally trying new things keeps the lives of the sexually woke interesting and vibrant. If life and sex are getting mundane and routine, it takes intention to change things. We are all creatures of habit, and changing routines is not instinctual. But according to the sexually woke, it's important. Going to the edges of our comfort zones—and beyond—is vital for growth, as we know to be true for any human activity. If you want to get better at running, you have to run faster and longer than your comfort zone dictates. To build muscle, you have to lift heavy things repetitively and literally break muscle down so it can rebuild.

I was at a spinning class the other day, and my instructor Meg challenged us to: "Push yourself to the point of doubt. If you are certain that you can do it, you are not trying hard enough. Go into a new world of uncertainty. That's where the growth is." Okay, so this is a spinning class, but one of the reasons we go to things like spinning class is to practice how to live when we are faced with challenges in our day-to-day life. We need to get comfortable with uncertainty if we are going to grow. Period. Why should sex be any different?

Remember, Elizabeth has been married for almost 30 years, but she still has a lot of fun trying new things:

> I'm going to be an empty nester. So I'm like okay, this is going to be a new day for our marriage. Last year, we went on a trip alone for the first time. In retrospect, I think you should have a date night or one weekend a month with your spouse, but believe it or not, we never did. We went on trips but always took the kids. So we decided to go to Cabo by ourselves. It was scary because I thought, 'Oh my God, I have never been alone with my husband for that many days. Are we still going to love each other?' I had butterflies in my stomach, but it turned out to be the most amazing experience of our lives. So we ended up buying a place in Cabo. Now it's like, 'When do I get to have you to myself again?'
>
> Now we love to go on dates. I want to look pretty and feel pretty. I want to be able to dress sexy and go out. Sometimes he will get there before me, and we will pretend we don't know each other. We do silly things like that, but they aren't silly. To keep the relationship exciting, there's the excitement of getting ready, of

being surprised like if I don't know where he's taking me tonight. Sometimes we will get a room at a hotel here in town just because.

One night he surprised me with dinner at a Spanish restaurant with Castilian Flamenco dancers. Right before the show, I needed to go to the bathroom, and I had a little black dress on. As I was going to the bathroom and my undies were down to my ankles, I thought, 'You know what? I don't even need these.' I put them in my hand, went back to the table, and gave them to him under the tablecloth. He nearly died. He questioned, 'You don't have any underwear on?' and I said, 'Nope.' It was on his mind the whole night. It's fun; I mean you have to make it fun.

For Alison it works like this:

We like to try different stuff because now we have plenty of time. We just enjoy each other. No one is at the house, and we can make noise. We try toys, and we try oils; we try this and that. We like to get online and shop together for fun sex toys. We were talking one day, and I said, 'So and so says they don't like sex.' He responded, 'Well, they are not doing it right!'

Victoria and her husband put time into educating themselves and reading books:

We read them together and talk about them, and he tried some different positions that would get more friction. Experimenting with different things was really exciting.

Keeping things fun and new are important to Daniella and Carl:

We're vocal, we talk to each other, and we share our fantasies during the moment. We like to get massages and bathe together. Sometimes we'll watch a little soft porn just to get things going. To see him excited turns me on and excites me. When we are feeling frisky, we egg each other on. It's a lot of fun. Now that the kids are all gone, we don't have to be quiet, and we don't have to lock the door. We can start to get excited when we're watching TV and then go to the bedroom. We can start being sexy at the restaurant and then come home and take our clothes off as we walk to the bedroom and not have to worry about who's listening or when the kids are coming home. 🙶

Jill and Adam enjoy every other weekend with no kids. There are pros and cons of joint custody, but one pro is that they have the ability to not worry about kids for a little while:

🙶 We are exploring together and learning new things about each other's bodies. Sometimes trying something new for us means not feeling pressure to 'finish' in the traditional sense. On a recent vacation, we massaged each other's shoulders, eyes closed, in a public hot tub at a hotel, and we both felt that it was one of the most intimate experiences we have ever had. 🙶

One thing that is universally valued by the sexually woke is growth. If you want to get the same result, do the same thing. To get a better result, try something different. It's as simple as that.

Speak Appreciation

Being intentional about appreciation and regularly making a point of it is a recurring theme of the sexually woke. Giving appreciation freely is an act of generosity, which if genuine, comes from a place of abundance. As discussed previously, living in a scarcity mindset makes it really hard to be generous. If I don't have enough for myself, it's not natural to give anything away. In this way being enough and giving appreciation go hand in hand. Alison remembers this well:

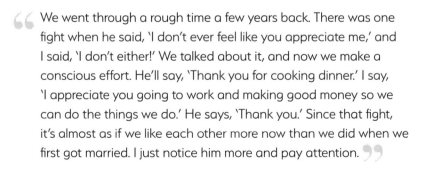

🙶 We went through a rough time a few years back. There was one fight when he said, 'I don't ever feel like you appreciate me,' and I said, 'I don't either!' We talked about it, and now we make a conscious effort. He'll say, 'Thank you for cooking dinner.' I say, 'I appreciate you going to work and making good money so we can do the things we do.' He says, 'Thank you.' Since that fight, it's almost as if we like each other more now than we did when we first got married. I just notice him more and pay attention. 🙶

Crystal is excited to share:

> My husband will still look at me and say, 'You're just so sexy.'
> I've put on a lot of weight since we got married. I'm a size 14. For
> me, because he thinks I am so awesome, I think that's sexy. He
> doesn't care about my weight. He really digs me and tells me that
> all the time. I'm sexy because he loves me. He doesn't take me for
> granted, and that's so attractive to me.

Daniella smiles and shares:

> Carl has always told me that I'm beautiful and is always attracted
> to me. If I'm naked, he'll say, 'Mmmm... You look great!' That kind of
> thing. So I've never felt jealous or insecure, and that makes him so
> attractive to me.

It's easy to say thank you or to give a compliment, and it means so
much. So why don't we do it more? That old programmed scarcity
mentality is a sneaky actor: Our ego feels like there is only so much good
to go around, so we better hold onto it and not give anything away. And
when we see the world like that, if we build someone else up, that makes
us feel small. Seeing this primitive and completely unhealthy behavior
for what it is and letting it go is a brave step to the left on the love-fear
spectrum.

A few years ago, I set an intention to always say something out loud
when I was thinking something positive about a person, whether it was
my partner, kids, or a stranger. I put this into action at a Starbucks® when
a rather grumpy-looking woman a few years older than me was in line
wearing a little tennis skirt. She had gorgeous legs. I looked at them in
awe. I could have let that thought pass, but instead I said, "Excuse me,
I just wanted to tell you that you have gorgeous legs." She immediately
lit up, and we talked for five minutes about her workout routine, her
mom's genes, and the products she uses. Before leaving, she said, "Thank
you. That made my day." I have no idea what she did differently that day
because of our interaction, but I like to think she treated people more
kindly and maybe even went home and made love to her husband.

When you think of appreciation, just say it. I challenge you to make
this an intention and a commitment.

Playtime

I love this dictionary definition of play: "to engage in activity for enjoyment and recreation rather than a serious or practical purpose." Many of us have forgotten how to play as adults. When did life get so serious? Personally, I was conditioned to think of most forms of play as a "waste of time." The understanding that doing nothing much and for no reason is one of my most valuable uses of time, has dramatically improved my own happiness and that of the people around me.

Intentionally spending playtime together is key to the sexually woke. As Veronica explains:

> I really think couples need to have fun together. One thing we connect with is dancing. When we dance, he leads, and I follow. That's sometimes a huge task. We had this awesome dance instructor, and the number one thing we had to learn was connection. If you don't hold each other right, your dance is going to be off.

Maria describes:

> We have such a connection that he doesn't watch any TV shows that we both like unless we're together. We do things together. We walk together. We like to travel together. He likes to play the piano, and he likes that I sit there with him and listen. We like gardening, and we like drinking wine. There's a real friendship. I don't want to have sex with someone who doesn't listen to what I have to say or doesn't do activities with me. To me, intimacy and having fun together are the flames that keep your relationship alive. Even if we are really busy, we find the time to cuddle together, go for a walk, or just do something to acknowledge each other and to talk and laugh about how our days went. That's what keeps our relationship where it is.

Daniella and Carl have "tennis Tuesday" and love to ride bikes and hike together:

> I like to ride behind him, then come up alongside him and tell him his butt looks good. He does the same for me. If we find a ping-pong table, we'll trash talk each other about who is going to win and do silly dances when we crush a point. We also love to travel together and have been on many, many long flights. Our ritual is to agree on a movie then count down 3-2-1 and start it at exactly the same time, so we can be watching it together on our tiny screens, holding hands. It's corny but fun. We want to share the same experience at the same time. It's connecting.

Use Words with Care

We all know that old childhood bully comeback: "Sticks and stones can break my bones, but names will never hurt me." Well that's just BS. Words can hurt a lot. Even in loving relationships, we can use words as weapons when we're triggered. When we know someone inside and out, we have enormous power to hit them with words in their most vulnerable spots. We know the one thing that our partner is most afraid or ashamed of and can fire that nuke if we ever want to. While the idea of wanting to emotionally destroy your partner with words seems ridiculous, people do it all the time. Wielding power and intentionally causing pain is a common tool in unhealthy relationships, but it's something the sexually woke never ever do.

Time and again in my interviews, the sexually woke shared ways in which they intentionally set habits around using kind words and peaceful conflict resolution. It's not that they never have conflict. In fact, they have plenty, but they resolve it with intention and kindness.

It took Elizabeth and Jake years to learn how to communicate well, but they persisted:

> All of this is maturity. It's not like I was born doing this right. You have to get it wrong before you get it right. Over time, you have to learn how to say what you mean and mean what you say but in a kind way. If you want to be happy, you have to be transparent about what you want, what you need, and be able to have a

difficult conversation. It's also important to know when it's not time to talk. If you are really worked up, you have to put a pause in it. 'I love you, but I'm not going to keep arguing right now. Tomorrow let's make a point to talk through this because my feelings are hurt.' Then you're free, and you aren't harboring all that resentment. If you are pissed off about something, and you aren't willing to voice it, then you are not going to even want to talk, let alone make love. It's like, 'Get away from me. I cannot stand you right now.' That's just not going to work.

And there are times when you just have to let things go. Those little three or four things that annoy you: are you going to focus on those or just let them go? Everyone has little idiosyncrasies. If they are not really impactful things, just let them go. Love people for who they are, and stop trying to change them. If it's a small thing, just let it go and stop bitching and nagging. "

Plenty has been written about the principles of Non-Violent Communication (NVC), a system developed by Marshall Rosenberg in the 1960s and followed by a book with the same name. While few had read the book, I found that many of the sexually woke were using these techniques. One of the key elements is using what is called "I" language which works for a few reasons. Beginning a sentence with "I feel ____" avoids putting the other person in a defensive mode. It feels like an accusation when the alternative "You make me ____" is used. Second, it is irrefutable. No one can argue with how you feel. It also avoids creating a "drama triangle" with its victim, villain, and hero. The pattern of NVC is to try some version of "I feel ____ when you do ____ because I need ____."

Yes, two people can form a drama triangle. It's pretty easy to assume two roles or even all three. I'm an expert at being both victim and hero in the same sentence. That might work something like this: "You make me so sad [he's the villain] when you change your plans at the last minute and leave me hanging [I'm the victim]. But I'll be just fine. I'm going to watch a chick flick [I'm the hero]." Can you imagine any way at all that this setup is going to end well? He now feels angry and annoyed, not to mention guilty. His choices are to leave and feel guilty or stay and feel resentful. Yuck.

See how much better this sounds: "Honey, is this a good time to talk?" (Get agreement first or wait until later.) "I feel hurt sometimes when you change your plans, and I think that's because I need to feel like I can depend on you. What do you think?" That's still a difficult conversation but much harder to argue with and much easier to work through. And it's coming from a place of possibility, honesty, and vulnerability, not from a place of passive aggression and victimhood. And since we are on the subject of sex, remember that no one wants to have sex when there is resentment in the air. Truly making love requires honest, kind communication.

Christina's advice to couples for communicating well, especially in the bedroom, is:

> I think the best advice I ever got was to say, 'I like it when you [blank].' You have to start with what you like. It's so positive, and men really want to know how to please you. If you don't tell them, how will they know? Instead of bitching about the things you don't like, start with what you do like. Be honest. Ask for what you want. I promise everyone is guessing, so don't keep them guessing. Wouldn't life be easier if we just said what we wanted? And it makes my husband so happy too.
>
> Now if something is wrong, I might say, 'I got my feelings hurt when you did [blank].' If I'm really upset, we are just to going to table it for a few days. Nothing good happens when we argue in that state.

Being intentional with our word choices to create harmony can come down to changing just one word, and the whole tone changes. Just like with changing the accusatory "you" to "I," the way we talk to ourselves can make a huge difference in our state of mind. A few years ago, my coach suggested I count how many times I say, "I have to," "I need to," and "I should." I followed this for a day and—wow—it was a lot! The invitation was to then change these words to "I want to" or "I choose to." Again, this simple shift moves us out of the victim position where everything is happening "to me" and puts us back in control of our lives. Elizabeth notes something similar and remarks:

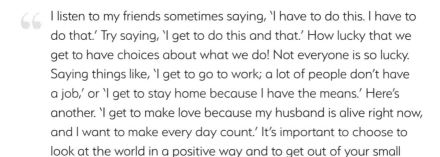

I listen to my friends sometimes saying, 'I have to do this. I have to do that.' Try saying, 'I get to do this and that.' How lucky that we get to have choices about what we do! Not everyone is so lucky. Saying things like, 'I get to go to work; a lot of people don't have a job,' or 'I get to stay home because I have the means.' Here's another. 'I get to make love because my husband is alive right now, and I want to make every day count.' It's important to choose to look at the world in a positive way and to get out of your small little world and see the big picture. If you can't do that, how are you going to have a close relationship?

It's Never Too Much

There's a joke I heard about a couple seeing a therapist. The wife complains, "He never tells me he loves me," to which the husband answers, "I told you I loved you when we got married 30 years ago, and I'll let you know if anything changes." The fact is humans need regular affirmation. It's hard to say I love you too much. Love is the gas that keeps that pilot light burning. Intention and attention guide the decisions we make to keep that love in our awareness.

For me, intention and attention equate with presence. When it comes down to it, the sexually woke were present—maybe not all the time but on some level they deeply understood its importance. If there is one thing I have learned from my own experience and this amazing research, it's that most of us are missing out on our lives by being somewhere else. As my teacher Vinny said:

I used to think that there was always something missing in my life. It turns out that the only thing missing was my presence.

Amen.

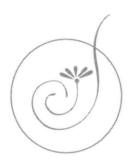

Final Thoughts

I think everything I've learned about midlife, sex, and relationships can be summed up in one sentence:

"Your task is not to seek for love, but merely to seek and find all the barriers within yourself that you have built against it."
—**Rumi**

The beautiful thing is that Rumi was a 13th century male Persian poet and mystic in the Sufi tradition. Now more than 800 years later, these words are just as true as they were then. Rumi wrote extensively about human love in the context of spirituality and has been a great resource for so many of us exploring these ideas. Transcending time, culture, and religion, he speaks to the core understandings of the sexually woke.

We are inherently perfect and lovable. Love and happiness need to be cultivated within first rather than seeking a fix from the outside. If we break down the walls of conditioning, we will exist in a field of nothing but love and connection. Wow.

Sometimes I think I've figured out something new, and then I realize nothing is new except how much you can see of what's always been there. I wish you all luck on this brave journey toward awakening.

With love and gratitude,

Dr. Susan

NOTES

INTRODUCTION

Chodron, Pema. *The Places That Scare You: a Guide to Fearlessness in Difficult Times*. Boston: Shambhala, 2018.

Comfort, Alex, and Susan Quilliam. *The Joy of Sex*. New York: Harmony Books, 2015.

Silverstein, Shel. *The Missing Piece Meets the Big O*. New York: Harper & Row, 1981.

PART 1

Brown, Brené. *Braving the Wilderness: the Quest for True Belonging and the Courage to Stand Alone*. 1st ed. New York: Random House, 2017.

Garrison Keillor. "Garrison Keillor Quotes." BrainyQuote, Xplore, http://www.brainyquote.com/quotes/garrison_keillor_137097.

"Glenn Close: 'You Don't Lose Your Sexuality as You Get Older'." *The Guardian*, Guardian News & Media (21 Jan. 2019): http://www.theguardian.com/film/2019/jan/21/glenn-close-the-wife-dont-lose-sexuality-as-get-older. Accessed 4 Feb. 2019.

Goodman, Michael P., et al. "Evaluation of Body Image and Sexual Satisfaction in Women Undergoing Female Genital Plastic/Cosmetic Surgery." *Aesthetic Surgery Journal*, vol. 36, no. 9, (15 Apr. 2016): pp. 1048–1057, doi:10.1093/asj/sjw061.

O'Donohue, John. "For a New Beginning." *The Value of Sparrows*, 12 Dec. 2012, http://thevalueofsparrows.com/2012/12/12/poetry-for-a-new-beginning-by-john-odonohue/.

Pinker, Steven. *The Better Angels of Our Nature: Why Violence Has Declined*. 1st ed. New York: Penguin Books, 2011.

Van Anders, Sari M, and Emily J Dunn. "Hormones and Behavior: Are Gonadal Steroids Linked with Orgasm Perceptions and Sexual Assertiveness in Women and Men?" Issue 2 ed., vol. 56, *Elsevier B.V.*, 2009, pp. 206–213.

PART 2

Ash, Mary Kay. *Miracles Happen*. New York: Harper Perennial, 2005.

Beattie, Melody. *Codependent No More: How to Stop Controlling Others and Start Caring for Yourself*. 1st ed. Center City, MN: Hazelden Publishing, 1986.

Brown, Brené. *Braving the Wilderness: the Quest for True Belonging and the Courage to Stand Alone*. 1st ed. New York: Random House, 2017.

Brown, Brené. *Daring Greatly: How the Courage to Be Vulnerable Transforms the Way We Live, Love, Parent, and Lead*. 1st ed. New York: Avery, 2012.

Crowe, Kelsey, and Emily McDowell. *There Is No Good Card for This: What to Say and Do When Life Is Scary, Awful, and Unfair to People You Love*. 1st ed. San Francisco: HarperOne, 2017.

Dalai Lama and Dennis Estrada. "Your Precious Human Life." *Your Precious Human Life*, 1 Jan. 2011, http://buddhistreflections.blogspot.com/2011/01/your-precious-human-life.html.

Descartes, René. *Discourse on Method ; and Meditations on First Philosophy*. Translated by Donald A. Cress. 4th ed. Indianapolis, IN: Hackett Classics, 1999.

Dethmer, Jim, et al. *The 15 Commitments of Conscious Leadership: A New Paradigm for Sustainable Success*. 1st ed. Dethmer, Chapman & Klemp, 2015.

Einstein, Albert, and Alice Calaprice. *The Ultimate Quotable Einstein*. Princeton: Princeton University Press, 2013.

Estrada, Dennis. "Your Precious Human Life." *Your Precious Human Life*, 21 Jan. 2011, http://buddhistreflections.blogspot.com/2011/01/your-precious-human-life.html.

Foster, Jeff. "Anger: The Extraordinary Fire Inside." Jeff Foster (http://ww.lifewithoutacentre.com), 16 Dec. 2018.

Hendricks, Gay, and Kathlyn Hendricks. *Conscious Loving Ever After: How to Create Thriving Relationships at Midlife and Beyond*. Reprint, Carlsbad, CA: Hay House Inc, 2016.

Holmes, Tom, et al. *Parts Work: An Illustrated Guide to Your Inner Life*. 4th ed. Kalamazoo, MI: Winged Heart Press, 2007.

"Introduction to Carl Jung – Individuation, the Persona, the Shadow and the Self." *Academy of Ideas*, 22 Mar. 2018.

Jung, C.G. "A Quote by C.G. Jung." Goodreads; Goodreads, http://www.goodreads.com/quotes/18322-one-does-not-become-enlightened-by-imagining-figures-of-light.

Kall, Rob. "Praise Allah, but First Tie Your Camel to a Post." *OpEdNews*, 5 Feb. 2010, 02:18:21, http://www.opednews.com/Quotations/Praise-Allah-but-first-tie-yo-by-Sufi-Saying-100204-272.html.

Mayle, Peter, and Arthur Robins. *What's Happening to Me?: the Answers to Some of the World's Most Embarrassing Questions*. New York: Lyle Stuart/Kensington Pub., 2001.

Mayler, Peter. *Where Did I Come From?* New York: Carol Pub., 1975.

"Matthew 10:39." *The Open Bible: New Living Translation*, Nashville: T. Nelson Publishers, 1998, pp. 1258–1258.

Neff, Kristin. "Compassion." *Self*, http://self-compassion.org/.

Nisker, Wes. *The Essential Crazy Wisdom*. Nook Book ed. Berkley: Random House, 2012.

Oliver, Mary. "The Summer Day," by Mary Oliver - Poem 133 | *Poetry 180: A Poem a Day for American High Schools*, Hosted by Billy Collins, U.S. Poet Laureate, 2001-2003 (Poetry and Literature, Library of Congress), http://www.loc.gov/poetry/180/133.html.

Peck, M. Scott. *The Road Less Traveled: a New Psychology of Love, Traditional Values and Spiritual Growth*. Anniversary ed. New York: Simon & Schuster, 2002.

"Poem: 'Clearing,' by Martha Postlewaite." *Compassionate San Antonio*, 10 Dec. 2018, http://sacompassion.net/poem-clearing-by-martha-postlewaite/.

Redfield, James. *The Celestine Prophecy: An Adventure* (Celestine Series, #1.). 1st ed. New York: Grand Central Publishing, 1993.

Robinson, Marnia. *Cupid's Poisoned Arrow: from Habit to Harmony in Sexual Relationships*. 1st ed. Berkley: North Atlantic Books, 2009.

Schwartz, Richard C., and Martha Sweeny. *Internal Family Systems Therapy*. 2nd ed. New York: The Guilford Press, 2019.

Sharma, Robin S. "A Quote by Robin S. Sharma." Goodreads; Goodreads, http://www.goodreads.com/quotes/534889-the-mind-is-a-wonderful-servant-but-a-terrible-master.

Siegel, Daniel J. *Mind: a Journey to the Heart of Being Human*. 1st ed. New York: W.W. Norton & Company, Independent Publishers since 1923, 2016.

Siegel, Daniel J. *Mindsight: The New Science of Personal Transformation*. 1st ed. New York: Bantam Books, 2010.

Silverstein, Shel. *The Missing Piece Meets the Big O*. New York: Harper & Row, 1981.

Sperry, Rod Meade. "'Right Now, It's Like This': How to Make This Popular Buddhist Phrase Work for You." *Lion's Roar*, 20 Apr. 2017, http://www.lionsroar.com/right-now-its-like-this/.

Stein, Garth. *The Art of Racing in the Rain: A Novel*. New York: HarperCollins, 2009.

Taranatha. *Steps to Happiness: Travelling from Depression and Addiction to the Buddhist Path*. Cambridge, UK: Windhorse Publications, 2006.

"The Conscious Leadership Group." *The Conscious Leadership Group*, http://conscious.is/.

"William Arthur Ward Quotes." BrainyQuote.com; BrainyMedia Inc, 2019. 17 December 2019. https://www.brainyquote.com/quotes/william_arthur_ward_190445

Zenji, Eihei Dogen. "Eihei Dogen Zenji, Author at *Tricycle: The Buddhist Review*." *Tricycle, The Buddhist Review*, 27 Aug. 2015, https://tricycle.org/author/eiheidogenzenji/.

PART 3

Nin, Anaïs. "A Quote by Anaïs Nin." Goodreads.com; Goodreads Inc., https://www.goodreads.com/quotes/2846-and-the-day-came-when-the-risk-to-remain-tight.

Rosenberg, Marshall B, and Deepak Choprah. *Nonviolent Communication: A Language of Life; Life-Changing Tools for Healthy Relationships*. 3rd ed. Encinitas, CA: Puddle Dancer Press, 2015.

Rumi. "A Quote by Rumi." Goodreads; Goodreads, Inc., https://www.goodreads.com/quotes/9726-your-task-is-not-to-seek-for-love-but-merely.

Zander, Rosamund Stone, and Benjamin Zander. *The Art of Possibility: Transforming Professional and Personal Life*. Reprint, New York: Penguin, 2002.

INDEX

ACKNOWLEDGMENTS

First and foremost, to the women who completed my study and shared the most intimate and candid moments of your lives with me, I cannot thank you enough. Your generosity will hopefully help so many women find what they have been looking for by seeing themselves through your stories. To Linda Gilbert at Ecofocus Worldwide, Lyn Ciocca McCaleb at What Matters Coaching, and Dale Engelken at Genesis Insights who helped to design and interpret the study, and to Ray Wolf my publishing agent for believing in a first-time author—I couldn't have done it without you. A huge thanks also to my editors and early readers Elizabeth Fordham, Alexis Latner, Kathryn Humphries, and Jonna Miller for your honest criticism and amazing eyes. And to my dear friends and former partners at Complete Women's Care Center who encouraged me and allowed me the time to write this book. I love you all.

I would also like to recognize some extremely important authors, speakers, and researchers who have shaped my life and this book, including Brené Brown, Tara Brach, Kristin Neff, Dan Siegel, Ben Zander and Gay, and Kathlyn Hendricks. To Jim Dethmer, Diana Chapman, and the Conscious Leadership Group, thanks for hanging in there with me and trusting in my potential. And to Erin Weed at EVOSO Academy, thanks for "digging me" and helping me find my message.

To the monks and residents at the Crestone Mountain Zen Center, thank you for sharing your space, support, and silence so that I could get this written. And to my friends and teachers Vinny Ferraro, Federica Clemente, Chris Crotty, Catherine Hansen, and MaryJo Rapini, you inspire me every day to show up as my best Self.

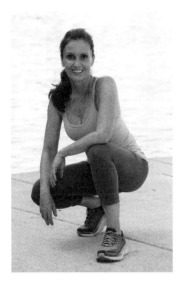

Susan Hardwick-Smith, M.D. is the Founder of Complete Midlife Wellness Center in Houston, TX, a concierge practice focusing on sexual and hormonal wellness. She recently retired as the Founding Partner and Medical Director of Complete Women's Care Center in Houston, one of the largest all-female OB/GYN groups in the United States. She is the recipient of multiple awards, including membership in the "Texas Super Doctors Hall of Fame," and has been voted one of the "Top 3 Rated Gynecologists" in Houston multiple times. She is also an International Coach Federation certified Executive Leadership Coach, as well as a Conscious Leadership instructor and practitioner, and has been a meditation student and teacher for many years.

Dr. Susan works as a volunteer surgeon in several African countries and serves on the Board of Child Legacy International in Malawi. She founded the AGIL Wellness anti-aging skincare and hormone supplement line to benefit women's health projects in rural Africa through the AGIL Foundation (www.AGILwellness.com).

As an experienced marathon runner and Ironman triathlete, she is passionate about fitness after 50 and the benefits of a plant-based diet for both personal and ecological health and longevity. Dr. Susan lives in Houston, Texas with her family of humans and animals.

www.DrSusan.com